"A book that must be handled with care."

— *Los Angeles Times*

"....not a cold, practical manual, though the information can be found in it."

— *The Lancet*

"It is the only guide to self-deliverance for the dying in the United States."

— *Arizona Daily Star*

"A more compassionate work than its British counterpart, Let Me Die gives case histories of desperately sick patients who have sought to end their lives. In recounting successful attempts, the book gives the precise doses of the drugs used."

— *Time Magazine*

"A restrained but highly graphic book detailing effective and relatively painless methods for 'delivering' the terminally ill from pain-wracked life to death."

— *San Francisco Examiner*

"The author of 'Jean's Way' has written another controversial book - a kind of do-it-yourself suicide manual for the terminally ill."

— *Chicago Tribune*

" 'Let Me Die' describes not only painless ways to end one's life. It deals with the kind of decisions someone facing such a prospect must make."

— *Philadelphia Bulletin*

D0974642

LET ME DIE BEFORE I WAKE

Hemlock's book of self-deliverance
for the dying.

Derek Humphry

Published by the Hemlock Society
Los Angeles
Distributed by the Grove Press
New York

Member's draft, 1981
First edition, 1982
Second edition, 1983
Third edition, 1984

ISBN Number 0-9606030-0-X
Library of Congress Number 81-80816

Published in the U.S.A. by
The Hemlock Society
P.O. Box 66218
Los Angeles
CA 90066

Printed in the U.S.A. by
Delta Lithograph Company
14731 Califa Street
Van Nuys, CA 91411

For all those who have
contributed to this book.

They have suffered, endured
and triumphed.

Origins and purposes

First editions of this book in 1981 were sold only to members of the Hemlock Society. The public demand for practical knowledge about voluntary euthanasia showed that the book had a wider audience, resulting in this improved and extended 1985 edition.

This book is not able to help those who are contemplating suicide because they are unhappy with life, or are suffering from a psychological affliction. It addresses the option of rational suicide only for a person in advance terminal illness or serious incurable physical illness.

A person contemplating deliberate self-destruction for any other reason should convey this intention to all or one of the following: Closest family or friend, physician, psychiatric counsellor, priest, or minister. If the intention remains, contact a Suicide Prevention Center (listed in telephone books, or ask hospitals). In some countries this type of counselling is done by the Samaritans.

Derek Humphry, Director of the Hemlock Society, was a newspaper reporter for 35 years, working for many British journals. He spent 14 years with the London *Sunday Times* where he began to write books on racial problems, policing and civil liberties. In 1978 he moved to the USA to work for the *Los Angeles Times.* The international acceptance of *Jean's Way,* the story of his first wife's death, as a classic account of rational voluntary euthanasia, launched him on a campaigning career for the right of self-deliverance. In 1980, in Los Angeles where he now lives, he and his second wife, Ann, formed the Hemlock Society, the first such group in North America.

CONTENTS

INTRODUCTION

Then is it sin
To rush into the secret house of death
Ere death dare come upon us?
—WILLIAM SHAKESPEARE

After *Jean's Way* was published in 1978, I was deluged with inquiries from all over the world from people who wanted to know what the poisonous substances were that my first wife had used to end her life after a long fight with bone cancer. These questions came, so far as I could tell, from people who were terminally ill and looking for information which would ensure them a graceful death if life became unbearable.

The police also wished to know the name and address of the physician who had given me the drugs which induced Jean's prompt loss of consciousness, to be followed by peaceful death within fifty minutes. They intended to prosecute him for supplying drugs to a non-patient. Nobody received an answer on this point. I told my correspondents, quite truthfully, that I did not know the brand names of the substances and, because of the public controversy raging around my case at the time, I did not dare ask the physician. Secretly, I was glad that I did not know, for how could I have, with good conscience, sent the fatal formula to people whose true medical and psychological condition I had no knowledge of? All I had were the pathetic cries for help.

And of course I did not tell the police who my doctor friend was. To this day his identity remains a secret. There was some general criticism of me, quite justified, that I was in the elite position of having such a knowledgeable friend and keeping his name to myself. But what are friends for if not to turn to in time of need, and subsequently protect?

As a compulsive writer of books, it became obvious to me just after *Jean's Way** was published that a book on methods of suicide for the terminally ill was required. Perhaps I should be the one to tackle it? The controversy surrounding my part in Jean's death, however, was propelling me into being a spokesman for voluntary euthanasia on several continents, and there was no time for further books. Also, it was too soon. Although the case for voluntary euthanasia has been discussed by philosophers for centuries, the excesses of modern medicine are only just beginning to bring the argument to the wider public consciousness.

For the next two years the controversy swirled around my case and others, causing interest in voluntary euthanasia societies around the world to intensify. Those of us who "went public" discovered that thousands of others could relate to the experience through a personal incident, compassion, or the wish to

---

* Hemlock can supply paperback copies of *Jean's Way* ($6)

1

control the manner of their own eventual death in a similar way.

Britain has always been the international leader on the topic of voluntary euthanasia. The British Voluntary Euthanasia Society was started in 1935. It has had a hand in promoting four Parliamentary bills intended to make planned death with medical aid possible—all unsuccessful— but each one succeeded in raising the level of medical, legal and public consciousness. By 1979 EXIT (as it was briefly known) had undergone a transfusion of younger members who canvassed among themselves the idea of a publication that would offer explicit guidance to the dying on how to accelerate their death if they so chose. EXIT announced in early 1980 that it intended to publish such a booklet.

Almost immediately a storm of controversy on the scale of the abortion debates in the 1960s and 1970s burst around EXIT. It was led by the news media, who asked with naive incredulity: ''Are you really going to tell people how to kill themselves?'' EXIT's leaders replied that they were, but that such a course of action was recommended only if a person was terminally ill and able rationally to consider this option. EXIT's justification was that until a law permitting voluntary euthanasia was passed (which would place responsibility to help primarily on physicians), people had no alternative but to take their dying into their own hands.

The media around the world stoked the rumpus, for better or worse; as a result, support for voluntary euthanasia societies swelled. From being the tiny, slightly cranky groups largely consisting of little old ladies who did not want to face a sick and vegetative old age, voluntary euthanasia groups now found that they were recruiting much younger people, even teenagers. Voluntary euthanasia became a vogue in colleges as a special topic in students' projects. Membership of EXIT, stagnant at around 3,000 for years, rocketed in months to more than 10,000. Its leaders replaced the heads of abortion and women's rights movements as national personalities on television.

As well as galvanizing right-to-die opponents, the proposed booklet served to polarize the internal arguments among supporters of euthanasia as well. If one believed in the concept, then why not issue proper instructions to adherents for its decent execution? Some older members within the movement disagreed. While they believed deeply in the principle of rational voluntary euthanasia and planned to use it for themselves, it was more than they could tolerate to make the option available to all.

The root of this distaste for such openness about voluntary euthanasia undoubtedly lies within the realm of modern man's horror of irrational suicide. Of course, most of us know of someone who has taken their life when it was preventable. Suicide for an emotional reason is always tragic, and almost always unnecessary. But suicide is endemic in mankind, and however much we regret it, it will not go away. And if we care so much, why do we not do more about prevention, such as teaching parents to recognize the signs of potential suicide in their children? The suicide rate in the Western world appears to be increasing steadily, according to the statistics, particularly among the youth.

The other side of the argument, however, will not disappear or retreat just because of our distaste for emotional suicide. Modern medicine does much to prolong lives, but the extension of life does not necessarily mean that it has extended its quality. Some people can accept a diminution of the things which make life worth living; others of us cannot. Pain control and the praiseworthy work of the hospice movement have made huge strides, but that benefit does not in any way negate the arguments for voluntary euthanasia. Additionally, something like one in five cases cared for in hospices (granted that they are so limited in beds that they take only the severest cases of suffering) still die a painful or uncomfortable death.

If leaders of the medical profession are appalled by the number of requests they are getting for assistance in voluntary euthanasia, they have only themselves to blame. The fearsome machinery which they have brought to their healing arts invokes a feeling of horror in many people, magnified by the television media with its obsession for hospital dramas. We are all grateful for technological aid which enhances one's chances of survival after a sudden illness or accident, but the thought of remaining hooked up to machines via tubes to our orifices is, for many, the abnegation of human dignity. To die in such a manner is unacceptable. Is it any wonder that people wish to explore the concepts of voluntary euthanasia?

After EXIT's announcement about their self-deliverance booklet, the storm surrounding it spread to America, which has two powerful organizations involved with the issues of a good death. EXIT asked the Society for the Right to Die if it intended to circulate the booklet. Subsequently there was a board meeting to debate this, and the overwhelming decision was that the society would not distribute *A Guide to Self-Deliverance,* as the booklet was called. Its board of directors unanimously concluded that responsible control of its distribution would be virtually impossible. Nevertheless, a statement was issued stating that the society respected the freedom of an individual with a terminal illness that had robbed him or her of a meaningful existence to make a decision about ending one's life. It was not entirely surprising, despite the society's title, that they declined to enter the controversy. To have done so might have hampered the good work that this New York-based group does in influencing the state governments to improve legislation on issues of dying and death.

Concern for Dying is a New York based organization with some 250,000 supporters which attempts to educate health and legal professionals about the complexities of dying. It also distributes millions of living wills to the public. Until 1978 this group was called the "Euthanasia Educational Council," but changed its name because it felt that modern advancement in pain control techniques made the case for euthanasia less tenable, and the paramount need was for education in order to protect the rights of the dying. Concern for Dying also felt that the word "euthanasia" has Nazi-like connotations, i.e., extermination of second-class citizens. (In fact, the Greek origin of the word means "good death.")

Concern for Dying (C.F.D.) discussed whether it ought to publish EXIT's booklet and categorically decided that it would not do so. (Had it distributed it, its support from various institutions would undoubtedly have vanished overnight.) In a considered statement issued later, C.F.D.'s leadership said that they feared that if voluntary euthanasia became an acceptable option for those people with irreversible illness who desired it, there was a danger that the elderly would eventually feel themselves obliged to hasten their departures from this world, (something not even the most rabid euthanasist has advocated; C.F.D.'s edict dismally presumes that most elderly people lack any sort of lust for life). Still, spokesmen conceded to those of their members who might disagree with its stance that there should be an "understanding, accepting attitude" to a decision reached by an individual with inalterable, intractable pain who opted for suicide.

As EXIT forged ahead in the Spring of 1980 in the face of internal and public (and by now international) controversy, it became obvious that such a piece of literature was not going to be available in North America. Yet thousands of Americans were writing London asking either to join EXIT or to buy the booklet—or both. (Coincidentally, sitting in my filing cabinet was a pile of letters from Americans who had read *Jean's Way* and had taken the trouble to write and say that this was the way of dying that they wished were they in a similar situation.) EXIT's booklet was not yet published in England or any other country, stalled by disputes within the group's executive committee and later by legal actions.

The evidence of the American applications to join EXIT, plus my own correspondence, indicated that a certain number—as yet unknown—of Americans believed in active voluntary euthanasia, or self-deliverance, as it is also known. (Euthanasists are repulsed by the label of "suicide" in lieu of active voluntary euthanasia, since suicide is correlated with irrational behavior. The term "self-deliverance" is a more accurate description of the act.)

While working on a book of an entirely different nature at my home in Los Angeles, where I now live with my second wife, Ann, I began to discuss whether I should launch a sister group to EXIT in the U.S.A. and use it to circulate *A Guide to Self-Deliverance.* Ann, as ever my mentor and moving spirit, declared that together we should start a voluntary euthanasia organization, and she already had a name for it: "Hemlock." A month later we called a meeting, or "think tank," of people in the Los Angeles area who were experts in issues concerned with dying. We put to them a position paper, with charter principles, for a society called Hemlock which would publicly support the concept of active voluntary euthanasia for the terminally ill.

This assembly of lawyers, doctors, psychiatrists, psychologists, pharmacologists, thanatologists, social workers, teachers, and writers all agreed that there was a need for a pressure group such as Hemlock, and, after much discussion and some polishing, the charter principles were accepted. But out of that group of some twenty "interested" people—whom I then asked to join Ann and me in launching Hemlock—only two, Gerry Larue and Dick Scott, said unequivocally that they would support us. The remainder declined, refusing to join even as private, unpublicized members, fearing that if it ever became known that they embraced the philosophy of voluntary euthanasia for the irreversibly ill, their professional standing would be severely compromised.

Baffled that these people, all secure and eminent in their fields, could simultaneously agree with us but be afraid to join, Ann and I left the home of Dick and Linda Scott, who had hosted the meeting, still determined to press on. On August 12, 1980, we called a press conference to announce the formation of the national organization called Hemlock, with Professor Larue as President and Mr. Scott as General Counsel, Ann as General Secretary and Treasurer, and myself as Director. We four were the sole members at that point. Asked by America's press corps about the strength of our support, I answered briefly and optimistically, "Growing."

Our antennae did not fail us. Support flowed in at the rate of 150 members a month, so that by the beginning of 1981, we had 850 paid members. As a great many of these were couples, the number was closer to 1,500 people. We were and are very much a minority group, but unquestionably a valid and cohesive segment of the huge spectrum of American public-interest groups. The predicted hositility from pro-life groups, the Catholic church and the Bible-Belt did not surface, and we have proceeded—with surprisingly few hindrances—to set up a viable group and produce this book on self-deliverance.

Why am I now producing a book for Hemlock's supporters when I would not answer my correspondents' requests for information two years ago? A fair question. Morally it is one thing to give advice on self-deliverance to an unknown individual, and quite another to dispense it to the entire membership of an organization whose members have paid a subscription because they embrace the philosophy of voluntary euthanasia. It is also against the law (see appendix) to give advice on methods of suicide to an *individual* who subsequently does end his or her own life, but it is not against the law to give information to people in general, especially when that group constitutes a bonafide minority, and when that information is culled from sources which are already in the public domain—for instance, bookstores and libraries.

Let Me Die Before I Wake is somewhat different from EXIT's publication. It also differs from the booklet produced by Scottish EXIT, *How to Die With Dignity,* which was published in September, 1980, after it became clear that the London voluntary euthanasia group had run into serious legal tangles with their version. Both these booklets are straightforward, nononsense guides to methods of bloodless and painless suicide. Each has several-hundred-word preambles warning readers about the careless use of self-deliverance, and each counsels people to be careful that they are doing the right thing—both from their own point of view and that of their families. The booklets contain the basic information that most people want: the lethal dosage of drugs.

How to Die With Dignity is given only to members of the Scottish group. *A Guide to Self-Deliverance* was withdrawn because a court case left its future in doubt. In 1983, a British Court ruled that *A Guide to Self-Deliverance* was not as a publication unlawful but sale to a person intending suicide with intent to aid that act might be found criminal by an English jury. (London Times Law Report, April 29, 1983. Queen's Bench Division.) Hemlock's book suffers no such restrictions, either by law or self-imposed, as it is protected by the First Amendment of the US Constitution permitting freedom of speech.

Both booklets have been an important breakthrough with a new genre. We in Hemlock admire the courage of the individuals involved who have defied their detractors and gone ahead with their publications. They have paved the way for Hemlock, for which we are grateful.

The thrust of Hemlock, under Gerald Larue's leadership, has been somewhat different from other voluntary euthanasia societies in that we believe that the preparation for dying involves more complex problems than the mere act of deliberately ending one's life. Hemlock stresses the personal, family, social and psychological factors which interplay with one's decision for self-deliverance and in the required support of those close to the dying person. It is a common weakness among euthanasia promotion groups that the leaders for the movement need no convincing; together they campaign for radical changes in the law, often assuming that the reasons behind their campaign are self-evident. Active support comes from people whose own experience with terminal illness makes them instant sympathizers, and it is easy to forget that the rest of the world may still be struggling with the concept. The cancer sufferer in Wyoming may not have as many relevant facts, books to read, or good minds with which to debate, as one exposed to the more worldly climate of London, New York, or Los Angeles.

Hemlock believes that the concept of active voluntary euthanasia for the terminally ill should be tackled on two levels: raising public consciousness so that the old taboos drop away and ethical standards are modernized; and ensuring that appropriate guides and information are available to ordinary people who face a terminal illness—either of their own or within the family. In such a huge nation as the U.S.A., personal counseling by Hemlock is virtually impossible, so by means of in-depth correspondence, informative newsletters, and books like *Jean's Way* and *Let Me Die Before I Wake,* we hope to help people come to grips with their individual problems.

This book is an attempt to examine the problems surrounding active voluntary euthanasia with realism, practicality and love.

Derek Humphry
Los Angeles, May, 1981
Updated, October 1984

CHAPTER ONE

*Why are so many people more readily appalled by an unnatural form
of dying than by an unnatural form of living?*

—NORMAN COUSINS

Everyone wishes to die well. Quickly, without pain, without anguish and sparing loved ones a protracted deathbed watch. Quite often this manner of death comes naturally from sudden heart failure or from collapse leading to a coma followed by a rapid end. But not always. The only way to be reasonably certain of a good death is to plan it, and plan, if at all possible, when one is still in good health.

The first step in the plan is to think about which manner of death is compatible with one's desires and moral beliefs. A devout person attached to a particular faith will want to follow the credo laid down by his or her religion. Fee-thinkers, on the other had, have to chart their own destiny using more subjective guidelines, so this little book hopes to show how others have handled their terminal stages of life. Some people have stumbled onto the manner of their exit from this world after trial and error; an unknown number have been fortunate to get it right the first time, while others have added to their suffering by failing to die successfully and have precipitated increased agony and frusration and helplessness. In this chapter we shall report an example of success. These are not the real names.

Sonia Hertz suffered from cancer for seven years. The disease started in the breast and she underwent a modified mastectomy. Radiation treatment and chemotherapy temporarily checked the disease and the side-effects were, luckily, not too severe. Sonia and her husband, Carl, however, both in their late fifties, realized that she was not likely to live into old age, and they both set out to achieve many of the things they had dreamed about doing before the disease became too advanced. Their two children were now grown, Carl was earning a good salary as a C.P.A., and they indulged themselves with travel, tracing their ancestors in Germany and visiting places which Carl had seen as a wartime airman. For five years after the first attack of cancer, Sonia lived a very full life, working for a gourmet magazine, playing golf and working in a small antique whop which she partly owned.

In the sixth year Sonia's condition worsened; the cancer appeared in her lymph nodes. She was put on different chemotherapies, and radiation treatment was intensified. She soon became paralyzed, however, (probably through a stroke) and was subsequently hospitalized. After a few months she was able to walk with difficulty and was well enough to go home although her movements were much more restricted: a nurse was needed to lift her in and out of her bed and bath. Within a couple of months the paralysis gradually disappeared, and Sonia attempted to return to a fairly normal life, driving around seeing friends in the afternoons, but generally taking life easy. She and Carl did some entertaining, and they gave their daughter a fine wedding in the garden of their home.

Sonia spoke of her feelings during those days of remission: "Everything was a little bit more special then. Life had a greater intensity for me. People I knew were more beautiful, and I was more appreciative of things done for me."

Then came another relapse. Doctors found that Sonia's cancer had spread to the lungs and skin and they altered the treatments, discharging her from the hospital after a few days. Trying not to show the depth and extent of her feelings to her family, Sonia was now seriously depressed, for she realized she could no longer deny the fact that she was going to die before very long. Although she found Carl was a loving and supportive husband, she was unable to discuss her imminent death with him. Sensing her depression, her son and daughter urged her to see a psychiatrist but she refused, arguing that her problems were purely physical. She was able to stagger about the house, bruising herself badly bumping into furniture and breaking several household objects she cherished.

"I know I can't live like this," she told friends. But they did not suspect what she was about to do.

One day when alone in the house Sonia filled the bath with cold water and took ten Dalmane sleeping capsules (each of 30 milligrams), washing them down with a small amount of whiskey and orange juice. She planned to plunge into the cold water and die from the combined effects of the benzodiazepine, drowning and hypothermia (low body temperature). But before Sonia could get to the bath she passed out, and as she collapsed she hit her head on the wall. She lay on the bathroom floor unconscious for quite a while but did not die because, of course, the ten Dalmane sleeping capsules were by no means a lethal dosage.[1]

Not long afterwards, her son, Gordon, unaware of her intentions, came home and found her lying on the bathroom floor. He called the paramedics, who rushed his mother to the hospital where doctors noticed that she was suffering from an overdose of drugs; they immediately pumped her stomach out. When, a few hours later, she recovered consciousness, she still intended to commit suicide.

"I remember thinking in the hospital that if I could get to the window I would jump out," she recalled later. "But my limbs wouldn't take me to the window."

The first caller at her bedside was Gordon. Sonia immediately criticized him for calling the paramedics.

"Why didn't you let me die?" she shouted. "I'm going to die soon anyway!"

---

1. Dalmane (Dalinane in Britain) is the brand name for flurazepam, which is a benzodiazepine. Dr. George Mair, in his booklet *How to Die With Dignity* (Scottish EXIT, Edinburgh, 1980) says on P. 29 that the suggested minimum lethal dose of flurazepam is 600 milligrams (600 mg), which would be twenty thirty-milligram capsules 20 x 30 mg.) although he says the capsules should only be used in conjunction with other methods of self-deliverance, such as hypothermia, drowning or gassing.

It was the first the young man knew that he had interfered with a suicide attempt. Asking his mother to forgive him, he began to cry beside her bed. By chance at this point a doctor came into the room and admonished Sonia, adding, "It's a good thing you didn't take enough tablets to kill yourself."

Gordon was extremely relieved that he had not, after all, thwarted his mother's wishes, because he considered that she had this right. Sonia was both pleased and surprised to have an ally. They forgave each other and embraced. Carl, on the other hand, was upset but kept his emotions under control, feeling ambivalent about Sonia's wish for early death by her own hand. He did not criticize his wife's actions except to say many times: "How could you think of leaving me without saying goodbye?"

Ironically, Sonia's suicide attempt galvanized her family into action. Whereas before they had been more attentive to her physical needs, now everybody's feelings were out in the open. The family discussed Sonia's right to die among themselves and while it did not produce any solutions, at least they now knew how the others felt.

"It's hard to share a decision to die with those you love." Sonia told a friend. "But now that the way I want to die is out in the open, we all feel better. My husband respects what I want to do but doesn't want to be any party to it. My son respects my decision entirely."

Sonia had another remission after her suicide attempt, and although she was extremely frail and slept poorly, she felt that life was still worth living. One consolation was the fact that her son decided it was his duty to remain at home: he could just as easily write his dissertation there while caring for his mother as at the university. In the meantime, Carl sought a therapist's help to help him cope with the family's problems and his own feelings.

A friend asked Sonia if she now regretted her suicide attempt. "No," she replied. "I was very bad, very low, and all my dignity had been taken away from me. It's been very nice having this extension, but I regret I didn't take the right dose last time. I've decided that it's important to me to regain some control over my own life. I want to choose my own way of dying in order to retain my dignity. This choice is not easy, but it is the only way that I can have peace of mind."

Sonia carried on for another year after the suicide attempt, still determined to end her life in a planned, orderly manner. By now she looked an extremely fragile, seriously ill person. One day she decided to ask her doctor if he would give her the right amount of pills to take her life. Although fully aware of the extent of her illness he flatly refused to help. She told one of her friends about this and was advised to attend the clinic at a time when her regular doctor was on vacation on the chance that his replacement might be more responsive.

Several weeks later Sonia put her request to the second physician—whom she had never met— and he listened attentively, at the same time studying her medical chart. Suddenly he excused himself and left the room, returning later with a bottle of tablets in his hand.

"There you are," he said, "I think that's what you want." Turning on his heel, he left the room.

Sonia picked up the bottle and saw that it contained sixty Seconal capsules, each 100 milligrams (mg.) Her eyes brimming with surprise and gratitude, she left the clinic for home.

Now that she had the means to take her own life, Sonia spent a few days quietly at home reviewing the situation.

"I'm getting so much weaker," she told her friend. "It's no fun living like this. My husband is darling, he'll take me anywhere, do anything for me, but I haven't the energy to go on. I'm getting so tired, I want out. This time my decision is based entirely on my physical condition, whereas last time it was because I was depressed at my physical condition. I'm thinking clearly now. It's been a long fight, and it's not fair to myself to go on any longer."

She was, however, deeply troubled about two things: how many of the Seconal should she take, and could she be sure that she would not vomit them? In addition, how could she be certain that her husband—who would remain at home when she took the overdose—would not be considered an accomplice in her suicide? For his part, Carl found it difficult to agree to any part in his wife's self-deliverance although, if she was going to commit suicide, he conceded that she should not be disturbed.

"I'm torn," he told a friend. "I agree with her right to do this. I agree with anybody's right to take their own life. I won't interfere. But I don't want any part of it."

Their daughter felt much the same. Only the son backed up his mother's right to end her life. It was Gordon, by chance, who helped resolve his father's conscience about assisting his wife in any way: he arranged for his mother to read a copy of *Jean's Way* and afterwards they left it lying around the house. They both noticed that Carl read it twice.

Soon Carl told Sonia: "I will help you." He did not explain why he had changed his mind, but it seemed to Sonia that because he had been able to relate to and identify with another man faced with a similar crisis, he could now see the importance of her own request to die well.

(Later Carl explained: "I saw parallels in the book to my own situation and things became clearer. Also, my son was strongly on his mother's side. Ever so gradually, Sonia persuaded me that it was my duty to help.")

Sonia told her husband that she was going to take entire responsibility for her actions. Her resolve was strengthened immeasurably by the Seconal she now had. A friend with some knowledge of drugs advised her that about two and a half grams (2.5 gm.) or twenty-five 100 milligram (25x100 mg.) tablets of Seconal would prove lethal, for such a tiny, very ill person as she was. While an empty stomach would facilitate absorption of the drugs, Sonia learned that vomiting would also be more likely. (Conversely, a heavy meal would slow down absorption considerably.) She decided to first take a travel sickness pill an hour before swallowing the Seconal, have a light snack a half hour later, and finally wash the drugs down with alcohol (which increases the drugs' lethality) and soda water (which whould hasten absorption). Having this knowledge gave Sonia a peace of mind which had previously eluded her. All she wanted from her husband was to have him present in the house to give her peace and security.

Sonia struggled on for a few weeks, gradually becoming weaker and increasingly troubled by the skin cancer. One Saturday she told Carl: "I think the time has come. I've had a very beautiful life. We've had thirty-seven good years together, you and I. I've had much pleasure out of life."

It was on that day Carl realized the crisis was coming, and he spent every moment with his wife, fixing an elaborate meal in the evening. Still troubled at her previous failure, Sonia kept talking about how she should take the Seconal and when.

Just before they went to sleep, Carl became a bit impatient with this dithering. He told her: "You must decide what to do and do it, or forget the whole thing. I just don't like this subject cropping up all the time. You can't do this to me."

Sonia apologized, took her normal sleeping pill, and dozed off. They woke up at the usual time Sunday morning and while Carl fixed breakfast Sonia waited in bed. Then she tottered weakly to the kitchen and drank a cup of tea and ate a piece of toast. Carl finished his breakfast and went to shave.

When he returned to the kitchen he found that Sonia had put the Seconal into a cup of tea and was trying with difficulty to drink it. Carl looked into the cup and saw a good deal of the powder still caked on the bottom. He did not think she had taken enough to provide a fatal dose.

Sonia said she was unwell and asked Carl to help her back to bed. He sat on the edge of the bed and they talked about how she felt. Carl was considerably agitated over the prospect of a second failure, knowing how much this would upset his wife, but Sonia told him to keep calm. They kissed and she fell asleep.

Carl wandered around the house, visiting the bedroom every few minutes, but saw that his wife was sleeping peacefully. After slightly less than an hour he noticed that she had stopped breathing. He called the paramedics and his doctor, all of whom assumed that she had died naturally from her cancer and never questioned the manner of her death.

Sonia had consumed only about one and a half grams (1.5 gm.) of Seconal, the minimum lethal dose,[2] but it was quite sufficient to end the life of a very sick, frail person who wished to die. Most people should take about 40 Seconal to be certain of self-deliverance.

---

2. See the toxicity chart of the thirty toxic drugs frequently used in suicide attempts in *The Prediction of Suicide,* edited by Drs. Beck, Resnick and Lettieri, (The Charles Press, Philadelphia, 1974).

11

CHAPTER TWO

Courage is the thing. All goes if courage goes.

—J.M. BARRIE

The stories in this chapter are about two brave and determined women. Each fought her illness until the end of life was in close sight, there was no realisti hope of further remissions and daily existence was painful and bleak in th extreme.

The first story is a condensed version of the book, *Jean's Way,* written b myself with the help of my second wife, Ann Wickett. Some details missing i the original have been added. It is perhaps helpful to point out two things abou this story: first, Jean had never considered the ethics of voluntary euthanasia I never once heard her mention the word, nor does it appear in that book. Neithe of us were members of any right-to-die group. The way she came to grips wit the problems of dying and the plan which she carried out with iron disciplin sprang from her instinct of what was right and best for her. Her request fo assistance from me seemed eminently reasonable, and, from the standpoint o having been her partner for twenty years, it was unthinkable that I should no cooperate.

Secondly, author though I was, I had no inkling of writing a book about Jean' dying until I was persuaded by Ann that not only was it a love story, but tha it had significance for other people too.

Many people ask me: What happened afterwards? It was not a secret in ou family that Jean had ended her life this way, and she had told quite a few friend of her intention. It was not until the book reached the bookstores three year later that the police began their inquiries. I doubt whether they would have acte at all had not so much controversy been stirred up by my story, causing severa members of the news media to ask the police what they intended to do abou a person who had so openly confessed to a crime. Immediately Britain's Direc tor of Public Prosecutions requested an investigation, which the detectives car ried out with considerable tact and intelligence. In response to their question I of course admitted my guilt,[3] but advised them that I would strongly contest be ing punished in court for my action.

The Public Prosecutor could not fail to hear the extensive public clamor ove the case—which even my worst enemies conceded tended on balance to favor

---

3. In England and Wales, although suicide itself is no longer an offense, a person wh aids, abets, counsels or procures the suicide of another is liable to a maximum penalt of fourteen years' imprisonment under Section Two of the Suicide Act, 1961. The con sent of the Director of Public Prosecutions to the institution of proceedings is alway required.

Jean's actions—and four months later he announced that he would not pursue any criminal charges on the grounds of "insufficient evidence." Needless to say the authorities had only my word that a "crime" had been committed. Jean was cremated the week after her death so only I knew that she had taken poison. As I refused to reveal the name of the physician who gave me the substance, the police could not verify that either.

What follows is a shortened version of the story:

Jean Humphry developed cancer when she was forty. At first, a mastectomy and radiation treatment arrested it temporarily, but the disease was particulary virulent. Within a year it had metastazised to the bone. Despite excellent medical treatment and many hospitalizations, Jean realized that she was going to die before long.

Five years earlier she had observed her mother's prolonged and agonizing death from cancer. The end for her mother came at home, with Jean and her father doing all the nursing. It was a painful and distressing illness, and Jean was both hurt and indignant that nothing had been done to help her mother die well. Most of all, Jean was concerned that no one in the family had forseen just how uncomfortable a death her mother would have. When her suffering was starkly in front of them, the indecision appalled Jean. Outraged at her mother's agony, she swore to herself that she would never let that happen again—either to the dying person or loved ones.

Now, unexpectedly, Jean was faced with her own impending death. At first she clung to life and struggled to postpone the end, moving home to a new location, starting her own small business and keeping up her involvement in politics, while at the same time being a committed mother and wife.

Eighteen months after the first detection of the cancer, however, she was so seriously ill that the doctors suggested to me she might have only a few days to live. To control the pain she had to be heavily dosed with narcotics which enabled her to sleep comfortably most of the time—otherwise she would have died from the sheer pain, one of her doctors noted. During one of her rare moments of consciousness she told the nursing staff that if she could not spend her days awake, then she did not want to live. A comatose existence repelled her, and she made this perfectly clear. As if challenged by this, the staff at the Churchill Hospital in Oxford, England, kept varying the pain-killing dosages until they found a formula which controlled the pain but left her in a greater state of consciousness.

The formula they were using is known as the Brompton Cocktail. Other names for this pain controller are Brompton Mixture, Brompton Solution and in America, generally Hospice Mix. The name "Brompton" comes from Brompton Hospital, London, where it was devised. In Britain the mixture consists of morphine, cocaine, alcohol (90 per cent), syrup and cholorform, with a phenothiazine to alleviate the effect of the morphine and to act as an antiemetic tranquilizer. In America, as cocaine is rarely used in medical practice, this ingredient is missing.

Within days this particular crisis had passed, and Jean's days were spent sitting up in bed, receiving visitors, and dozing. In her wakeful moments she was plotting a course of action which she revealed when I arrived at the hospital as usual one afternoon. After we had greeted one another and exchanged scraps of news, Jean made an obvious effort to pull herself together, indicating to me that there was something important she wished to say.

"Derek," she said, taking a deep breath. "I simply don't want to go on living like this. It's been pretty bad this week and I want you to do something for me. I want you to do something for me so that if I decide I want to die, I can do it on my own terms and exactly when I choose. The one thing that worries me is that I won't be in any position to make the right decision, what with my being knocked senseless by all these drugs. I might be too daft to know whether I'm doing the right thing or not, but I shall have a good idea when I've had enough of the pain. So I want you to promise me that when I ask you if this is the right time to kill myself, you will give me an honest answer one way or another and we must understand, both you and I, that I'll do it right at that very moment. You won't question my right and you will give me the means to do it."

I considered for a moment and answered, "If our positions were reversed, I know I would make the same request. I'll do whatever you ask.."

Jean was anxious that there should be no misunderstandings and wanted the pact to be crystal clear. "Do you promise that when I ask the question, 'Is this the end?' that you will give me the answer and then the means to carry it out?"

"Yes," I replied, taking both her hands in mine. "I promise, my darling."

Not long afterward Jean was well enough to go home, although most of the time she was too weak to leave her bed. She had sensed when the ambulance drivers carried her inside the house that this was probably her final homecoming. Yet despite the gradual deterioration of her body, her emotional strength remained constant, clearly reinforced by the knowledge that the manner of her dying would be both within her control and that it would not be painful. In a restricted way, her existence remained useful and extremely meaningful to her; she ran her life from her bed, communicated frequently with close friends on the telephone and helped others with their own problems at the same time.

Nine months after the making of the pact, her condition worsened dramatically. I realized that the time was imminent to implement my part of the bargain: getting the drugs which would help her die speedily. I had an instinctive feeling that it would be wrong to ask the doctors who had cared for Jean so well to help her die. Also, they might well refuse and somehow interfere with the carrying out of the pact. Luckily, I had known a physician practicing in Harley Street for years, and I decided to ask him for help. We met in his office one afternoon, and I told him all the details of Jean's medical situation and the manner in which she wished to die.

"I doubt if there is any decent existence left for her," the physician said," and I wouldn't blame you in the least if you wanted to save her any more pain and anguish."

As though it were an everyday occurrence, the doctor telephoned a pharmacist he knew at a local hospital and asked him what was the best combination of prescription drugs to end a life rapidly. When the telephone call ended, the doctor went to his drugs cabinet and mixed thirty (30) 100 milligram (mg.)[4] Seconal capsules with thirty (30) Codeine tablets[5] in a small bottle and gave them to me. He suggested that they be dissolved in water (at the last minute), although even then a bitter taste would not make them easy to drink.

I was still worried about how the end would come. By now Jean was in such a state of decline, with intense pain only relieved by massive drug dosages, that I considered that it would be kinder to just quietly slip her the overdose as a normal medication and allow her to die peacefully in the night. But the amount which had to be taken, together with the bitter taste, did not allow me to seriously contemplate this. It would have to be a mutual act, sanctioned by both of us.

A few days later the doctors examined Jean again. They found the cancer had spread through most of her bones and was affecting the lungs and kidneys; she was also developing thrombosis. Throughout her illness the consultant had repeatedly used the phrase: "We've a long way to go yet." Yet at this particular examination Jean turned to him and asked his opinion. "There's nothing more I can do," he responded honestly.

"Then let's give up trying and let me go home to die," she said. "I haven't the strength to fight any more."

She returned home by ambulance and for the next two days was quietly contemplative, placid and gentle, as though a state of grace emanated from her. I was aware that the part I was obliged to play in her death was about to be realized. Emptying the drugs out of their capsules into water, I stored them in a little bottle nearby.[6] My worst fear was that Jean, who adamantly refused to be

---

4. "The potential fatal dose of secobarbital (Seconal) is two to three grams (2 to 3 gm.), "*The Pharmacological Basis of Therapeutics,* by Goodman and Gilman, 6th edition, (Macmillan, New York, 1980), p. 359.

5. "Lethal dose (of Codeine) is about one-half to one gram (0.5 to 1.0 gm.)": *Clinical Toxicology of Commercial Products,* by Gosselin, Hodge, Smith and Gleason, 4th edition, (Williams and Wilkins, Baltimore, 1979), Section II, p. 159. Codeine has been in use as a pain-killer since 1886. James Long, in *The Essential Guide to Prescription Drugs* (Harper and Row, New York, 1980) notes on p. 169: "Codeine can increase the effects of all sedatives, analgesics, sleep-inducing drugs, tranquilizers, antidepressants, and other narcotic drugs."

6. Some doctors argue that diluting the pills' contents in advance can diminish the drugs' potency; had I been forewarned, I would have waited until the very last minute, although, fortunately, the brew still proved lethal.

put on a bedpan, would break limbs as she walked to the bathroom. Already her ribs—fragile and brittle from the advanced stages of the disease—had been broken in a minor accident. If further bones broke, I was sure she would ask for the overdose rather than be taken back to the hospital, where she would surely die. She did not hate hospitals and had always coped with them rather well, but her deepest wish was to die at home, which was the mirror of her lifestyle, and with her loved ones close by.

On Easter Saturday, March 29, 1975, Jean awoke in great pain, not an unusual occurrence, and, after she had taken medication, was able to sit up with the aid of pillows. She was quiet and serene, and when asked what she would like for breakfast replied that she wanted tea and toast as usual. When both she and I had finished our breakfasts, we sat looking through the picture window into the garden.

"Derek?" Jean called softly.

"Yes, darling."

"Is this the day?"

I needed a moment to control my emotions before I could say, "Yes, my darling, it is."

"How shall it be?" asked Jean. "You promised me you would get me something."

I said that the doctor friend in London had given me something which was quite lethal. "You have only to take this, and that is the end."

After a few quiet moments, Jean spoke again. "I shall die at one o'clock," she said. "You must give me the overdose and then go into the garden and not return for an hour. We will say our last goodbye here, but I don't want you to actually see me die."

We spent an emotionally-charged morning together talking and holding each other. At one point Jean applied her makeup and lipstick, tidied up her sidetables, and gave me instructions about what to do with her clothing and personal effects. We discussed the ups and downs of our twenty-one years of married life together, what would happen to our three sons, now in their late teens, and how I should handle my life afterwards. Jean kept reminding me of my promise to remarry whenever I felt like doing so.

A further instruction from Jean was for me to see her father after her death. "Tell him exactly how I died," she said. "I don't want him to think I died in pain or like a vegetable. He suffered enough when Mother died because no one would make any decisions. I want him to be sure to know I died this way."

We chatted on until Jean pointed out that it was ten minutes before one o'clock. I left the room, mixed the drugs into a cup of coffee and returned to her bedside.

"Is that it?" she asked. I nodded.

I took her in my arms and kissed her.

"Goodbye, my love."

"Goodbye, darling."

16

Jean lifted the mug and gulped down the contents completely, anxious not to leave any residue in the mug. The drugs took immediate effect, for she leaned back on her pillow, closing her eyes and falling fast asleep. Soon her breathing became slow and heavy.

I was afraid to leave her and ignored her request to go into the garden. I feared the drugs might not work and could not bear the thought that Jean might wake up and find herself alone and still alive. I had resolved that if the overdose did not end her life I would smother her. The thought of her coming round after so well-prepared a death and such a doughty battle against cancer was not something I could tolerate. I had been asked for help and, if it failed, I was obliged to go one step further and perform a mercy killing. When Jean vomited slightly I worried that she had lost too much of the Seconal and Codeine, but the light meal she had at breakfast helped the ingestion of sufficient drugs so that, despite the vomiting, her respiratory system was seriously depressed. Jean breathed heavily and noisily for fifty minutes and then died as I sat watching.

Mrs. June Spencer-Churchill was a little-known member of a famous English family, but the manner of her death earned extensive headlines and a good deal of controversy in July, 1980.

Aged fifty-seven at the time of her death, she was the widow of Randolph Churchill, the son of Winston. She had developed cancer fourteen years previously and at that time had had a mastectomy. After a long remission, the cancer spread through her body to her neck, spine, legs and other breast. Doctors told her that she faced paralysis prior to death and that there was nothing more they could do for her. her reply was that she would not accept the paralysis because it would cost her her independence. Doctors were sympathetic because Mrs. Spencer-Churchill's cancer was so severe that even with the use of heroin, the pain could not be completely controlled.

Within days after receiving the news of the certain prospect of paralysis, Mrs. Spencer-Churchill discharged herself from the Royal Marsden Hospital in West London and went home. She told a friend of hers that she had no intention of dying in agony but stopped short of telling him what she meant to do.

Sometime previously Mrs. Spencer-Churchill had joined the British voluntary euthanasia society, and had obviously thought a good deal about self-deliverance. Her apartment in Cornwall Gardens, Kensington, was no more than a good walk from the V.E.S. office. She read all the literature on voluntary euthanasia that she could find.

The day after leaving the hospital Mrs. Spencer-Churchill made the decision to end her life. She put a note on her apartment door telling her maid, Rosa, not to disturb her in the morning, and went to bed. She took the heroin[7] tablets

---

7. "In a nontolerant adult (i.e. a nonaddict), six one-hundredths of a gram (0.06 gm) (of heroin) is thought to be lethal. Not found in any legitimate product in the U.S.A." *Clinical Toxicology of Commercial Products,* Section II, p. 159.

which the hospital had given her for pain, and the Seconal prescribed to help her sleep. She drank a bottle of gin as she sat in bed, and then took one further decisive action to ensure her death.

She placed a platic bag (approximately three feet in length and one and a half feet wide) over her head and secured it with large elastic bands which tightly secured the bag. This had the effect, not of suffocating her, but of preventing the supply of fresh oxygen from reaching the blood. The drugs and alcohol she took ensured that she would lapse into a coma before the plastic bag could have its full effect, reducing any discomfort due to lack of oxygen. Precisely how many heroin and Seconal tablets Mrs. Spencer-Churchill consumed is not known, but the gin she drank undoubtedly doubled the drugs' lethality.[7] Using a plastic bag is undoubtedly a wise "fail-safe" technique, but the procedure is repugnant to some people.

Recording a verdict of suicide, the coroner said: "Mrs. Spencer-Churchill knew she was riddled with cancer in her bones, causing pain which was not completely controlled. The cancer had gone throughout her body and in time she would have been totally paralyzed and still in pain. It would seem to me that she died before she became totally dependent on others—something she couldn't bear."

Special Footnote:

Dosage Equivalents (not 100% equal)

1 gram (g) =	1000 Milligrams (mg) =	15 grains (gr)
0.5 g =	500 mg =	7½ gr
0.25 g =	250 mg =	3¾ gr
1 grain (gr) =	60 milligrams (mg) or 65 mg	
½ gr =	30 mg	¾ gr = 50 mg
¼ gr =	15 mg	3/8
gr =	25 mg	
1½ gr =	100 mg	

CHAPTER THREE

Be absolute for death; either death or life
Shall thereby be the sweeter.

—WILLIAM SHAKESPEARE

Alan Thomas was a comfortably-off building contractor in California. He had moved from the Midwest after serving in the war and establishing his own business, and sometime afterwards he and his bride, Ruth, started a family. Alan never revealed any religious beliefs and his wife had dropped her early religious fervor. Typical of a self-made man, Alan was a conservative Republican in politics, but he was never politically active or strident. The Thomases were a self-contained and self-confident family: such was the strength of their family bond and their adequate financial resources that when Ruth's sister became an alcoholic, they took in her three children and raised them along with their two daughters and one son.

Friends speak of Alan Thomas (not his real name) as a calm, strong man in his family life, while at work he was on as good terms with his carpenters as he was his wealthy and powerful clients. From home-building he had gradually switched to the construction of hospitals and dental clinics. When Alan and Ruth were in their fifties, the children, now grown, drifted away into careers and marriages, and the senior Thomases began to enjoy the fruits of their life's work. They became passionate golfers and travellers, and loved nothing better than to spend winters in Hawaii where they could play golf continually and enjoy the warm climate.

By the mid 1970's Ruth had what she told friends was "a spectacularly good marriage" with six "outstanding" children and ten "beautiful" grandchildren. Their cup of life was full, and deservedly so.

Without any warning, however, illness struck Alan in 1978 at the age of fifty-eight. All of his life he had enjoyed excellent health, and the sudden collapse was a blow to them both. Prior to spotting the first danger signals, Alan and Ruth were planning a cruise of the Caribbean in a chartered yacht in April, but when Alan noticed traces of blood in his semen he went for a check-up with an urologist. He drove himself to the hospital, alone, but came out a few weeks later a sick man. The outlook was bleak: cancer of the prostate which had already metastasized to the bone, appearing in his lower back and shoulder. There was also carcinoma in his bladder.

Pain started almost immediately, although not because of the disease: unfortunately an orthopedic surgeon had hit a nerve while making an injection. During the same treatment a blood vessel was also damaged, causing a massive hematoma (blood congestion) which had to be operated upon. Within a month of Alan's entering the hospital, the Thomases realized that the odds in favor of his recovery were remote, and they each began to think very carefully about what lay ahead for them.

Luckily money was not a concern, for in 1974 the couple had taken out a "catastrophe" insurance policy which covered everything up to three million dollars, with a $10,000 deductible. The premium was only $230 a year. Because of the enormous rise in health-care costs, Alan's illness cost the insurance company a small fortune, and the $10,000 deductible was an expense the Thomases could absorb fairly easily. It is difficult, almost impossible, to get such an insurance policy today on similar terms.

The total cost of Alan Thomas's treatments, both in and out of the hospital, was $69,500 (of which he paid the $10,000 deductible). The figure was provided by his daughter Carol, an accountant, who kept a careful log of the expense of her father's illness over the two years and four months that it lasted.

For the next five months Alan was in and out of the hospital for biopsies, checks, surgery, radiation and physical therapy. A neurologist struggled to relieve the terrible pain in the legs which had been caused by the clumsy needle, but there was still enormous discomfort.

In the space of a few weeks, Alan changed from a happy, outgoing man, into someone more reserved and cynical. On the surface he complained very little, still enjoying his evening cocktails with Ruth, and there were moments of pleasure despite the debilitating battle against the cancer and the pain. But the fact that he could not do things such as stand up long enough to pour a drink for his wife maddened him. Rather than provoke others with his anger he became withdrawn, as if he did not want anyone else to have to suffer too much along with him.

Because Ruth and Alan had always shared their problems, they now began to talk openly and in great detail about the future. One night after they had gone to bed Alan spoke very pointedly of his feelings. He told Ruth that he had no intention of ever reaching the stage where he was a vegetable, where he could no longer enjoy life, and where he would be a burden to everyone. As soon as that stage approached, he said, he wanted to die: "I don't want to go on to the end. I want to be able to take my own life. I don't want to do it in any way that is at all messy or would cause any grief to anyone. I just want to go to sleep."

Coincidentally, at the onset of Alan's illness, a neighbor suffering for a long time from acute emphysema shot himself in his shower. It had a profound effect on Alan. That evening he alluded to the incident again, mentioning to Ruth that he respected their neighbor's strength in finding a solution to his problem.

The dilemma they faced was not knowing exactly how long Alan could go on without unbearable pain and suffering. He was not suicidal and wanted to live as long as possible. But when would the final stages come? Both he and Ruth resolved to learn all they could about his condition before coming to any firm decisions. Ruth, devastated by thoughts of life without her husband, told Alan that when the time came for him to take his own life she intended to commit suicide too.

"I meant it very sincerely," she recalls now. "Alan was my life, and I couldn't

20

imagine life without him. But, my, he got upset at that! He talked to one doctor who was a friend and wanted him to talk me out of it. The doctor did so, but I told him that I had only threatened this to stop Alan from taking his own life. That wasn't actually true, but I resented having to talk to the doctor even though he was my gynecologist, about a matter which was between husband and wife. It was too private. I meant to die with Alan. We discussed it on a number of occasions in bed at night. Alan said that if I intended to do that, then he would not take his own life but struggle to the end and die whichever way was his fate.''

The topic was shelved during 1979 when Alan had some very good times, including a rousing birthday party given to him by his sons and daughters. He was able to get around either in a wheelchair or on crutches, and he and Ruth made their usual pilgrimages to the Hawaiian golf courses where he sat and watched Ruth play. Yet his health continued to deteriorate. Months later he underwent an orchidotomy (removal of the testicles) to try to stop the cancer from coursing through his reproductive system. He also underwent a series of chemotherapy treatments, and in September he nearly died of pneumonia.

During this time Alan's impending death was often discussed. He was a methodical man and wanted to die with his financial and legal affairs perfectly in order. He arranged that his death taxes would be at a minimum and that there would be cash in the bank to pay for the dues. On his last visit to Hawaii he leased a condominium for the following year. "It will be for you to come and enjoy yourself after I'm gone," he told Ruth with a smile. The golden moments were becoming fewer and fewer.

Months before he died, Alan said he wanted to do two things: take a ride in a balloon and make the arrangements for his own funeral. The family fixed the balloon ride, and by an odd chance the balloonist was also a funeral director. He and Alan got along well, so arrangements were made for them to meet in a few days. Ruth drove her husband down to the funeral home, and when Alan could not get out of the car the director came and sat with them. Alan quizzed him closely about funeral and burial practices and then he said that he did not want a service. Under the G.I. Bill, the government pays $450 towards an ex-servicemans's funeral, and Alan instructed him not to spend one dollar more than the government allowance. He wished to be cremated and have his ashes scattered over the Pacific Ocean.

Ruth was nonplussed by her husband's cool and premeditated approach to his funeral.

"Don't be shocked," he told her. "This is what I want. A year after I'm dead, when everybody's emotions are under control, have a party. Funerals are barbaric."

In April of 1980, Alan again developed pneumonia and was taken to the hospital. He was brought home after a week, and two L.V.N.'s (licensed vocational nurses) were hired to care for him daily. By this time Ruth was seriously underweight, suffering from insomnia and exhaustion. One evening after the nurse had gone home and it was cocktail time, Alan told Ruth: "I want to talk to you. Go fix us our drinks first."

As she got him his bourbon, she realized what was coming and, returning with the drinks, she sat nervously on the edge of his bed.

"We've got to talk about this dying business," he said. "If you are going to kill yourself, I'm not going to commit suicide. I'll go on to the bitter end."

Such an ultimatum disconcerted Ruth; she knew her husband would endure anything, making himself terribly miserable, just to keep her alive. Reluctantly she promised him that she would not end her own life.

"The way he put it to me, I felt that there was no other way I could do this," she recalls. "I didn't want to see him go through the agony, the degradation and everything else. I promised him that I would live."

Alan told her that she might even get married again. That made her mad. He gently reminded her of her duty to the children and their grandchildren. They went on to discuss the methods by which Alan could die peacefully. He had always assumed that he would take a handful of sleeping pills. Now he was faced with the problem of how many he needed to ensure lethality and which sort to use. There were plenty of tablets around the house, but he wanted to be certain of the right dosage.

Two years had passed since their first discussion of Alan's intended self-deliverance, and their conversation this time was much more emotional. Ruth promised that she would help her husband and that she would not take her own life afterwards. As they talked they held each other and wept until they were exhausted. Now that the decision had been made, Ruth made Alan promise not to end his life without telling her first, not wanting to experience the shock of suddenly finding him dead. It was to be a decision they would carry out together.

By this time Alan's pain was so severe that he was having regular injections of morphine three times a day. A doctor suggested that he have an operation to have his pituitary gland removed in the hopes that its absence would inhibit the pain. Anxious to clutch at any straw that would give him and Ruth a few more months together, Alan agreed. The operation stopped the pain for twenty-four hours, and then it returned as intense and blinding as it had ever been. A few days later Alan lapsed into a coma, but he was brought round in the intensive care unit of the hospital. After regaining consciousness, he returned home for the last time.

"I still had reservations about his suicide," Ruth said later, "I blame this on my very strict Episcopalian upbringing, and yet I knew it was the only thing for him to do. Still, it was uncomfortable to me. I didn't like the sound of it. But I would have done it right along with him without any qualms. What disturbed me most was the thought of being apart from him."

The gynecologist who was also a family friend asked Ruth why she had taken Alan to the hospital. "If you hadn't brought him in, he would have died," he said. "It would have been a blessing."

His statement unsettled Ruth and made her feel terribly guilty. She had in fact panicked when Alan went into the sudden coma and had rushed him to the hospital. (The coma was probably caused by the lack of cortisone. The necessary amount of cortisone needed by the body is produced by the adrenal gland under pituitary gland control, and Alan had been taking cortisone tablets to replace the gland's function. He had, however, chosen to stop taking them a week earlier.)

The gynecologist also told Alan the same thing: that if he had not come into the hospital, he would have died. "I think it was a mistake to bring you in here," he added.

This made Ruth furious. "I could have kicked him. He had no right to say it. My gynecologist had no right to interfere in husband and wife business. It was a tactless remark, but because he's a friend, I have since forgiven him."

This incident triggered Alan's resolve and helped him acknowledge that the time had finally come. He told his daughter Carol, "I can't go on putting everybody through this any more. I thought stopping the cortisone would do it."

The cancer had by now spread to the cranium, thus precipitating additional damage to the nervous system and affecting his behavior. He often hallucinated, and he sometimes lost control of his speech. The inability to speak properly infuriated him because he was always a very controlled man.

"Goddamn it! I can't even talk now!" he exploded, when he was unable to express what he felt.

One morning not long after this, Ruth spoke with her daughter Carol about the extent of Alan's illness. They were at a restaurant where Ruth was taking a brief respite from her nursing chores. Both she and Carol agreed that the end was very close, and when they returned home, they observed Alan drifting in and out of consciousness. The two women tried to talk to him in his occasional lucid moment. Suddenly he said very clearly, "I think we should send for Sam. I want Sam to come now." He was referring to a friend who was a radiologist who was well acquainted with Alan's medical history. The two men had been golf partners for many years.

Both Ruth and Carol realized that Alan's comment signalled the end. There was no doubt in either of their minds that he should die then, when he wished and when they were prepared to carry out his wishes. Acknowledging that they would go along with his requests, initially they intended to administer the existing supply of morphine solution. However, it was clear that the solution was too weak and the syringes too small to bring about a quick and effective death. Alan had obviously realized this problem, which was why he suggested that they contact Sam Browning for further help.

As soon as Ruth reached Dr. Browning, she told him of Alan's grave state and what she and Alan wanted done. Without hesitation, he agreed to help. When he arrived at the Thomas home, he found Alan fuzzy so that as he began administering the excessive doses of morphine, he was unsure whether Alan was aware of what was going on. While injecting, Browning had only a one (1) c.c. syringe to work with, smaller than he would have wished. A further difficulty lay in the fact that Alan's veins were difficult to find; Browning labored to administer a lethal dose of the drug, urging Ruth and Carol to massage Alan's body continuously to stimulate the dying man's circulation; otherwise the morphine would not be properly absorbed into Alan's system. Finally the last injection was given, and Browning advised the two Thomas women to wait and watch. "That's all I can do for now," he told them. "Let me know what happens."

Not long after Dr. Browning left, Alan regained consciousness and was lucid enough to ask for a drink. Carol brought him his favorite, bourbon on the rocks. With his arms around her, he told his wife: "Tomorrow I want you to go and play golf." Soon after that he lapsed back into a coma.

Around four o'clock Dr. Browning returned and gave Alan further injections. As he was about to administer the first shot, he murmured, "Alan, this won't hurt at all, old man." Alan opened his eyes, looked up at Browning, and then he winked.

"That wink was the communication between Alan and me," Browning recalls. "I said to myself, 'I could have talked to him, but it's too late.' I could have said to him, 'I'm saying goodbye.' I would like to have said that. But when Alan looked up at me and winked, I felt so much better because I knew that this was O.K. with Alan as well as with me, with God, with Ruth and with everybody."

Altogether Dr. Browning gave Alan nearly two dozen injections each of a quarter of a grain of morphine solution.[8] Alan, who had been taking one (1) c.c. injections three times a day as his normal pain-killing medication, had probably built up a tolerance to the narcotic. Thus his death was more prolonged than any of them would have wished.

Before he lapsed into a final coma from the effects of the second set of injections, Alan and Ruth kissed goodbye. Alan whispered, "I love you. I'll be waiting for you."

Ruth told him: "I've got so many things to tell you. I've not finished...Goodbye."

He lived for another nine hours, breathing slowly and heavily, which his wife and daughters found extremely distressing. (The younger daughter, Hilary, had joined them in the afternoon.) The end finally came towards 1:30 a.m. on Sunday morning, some twelve hours after the initial injection.

Ruth and her daughters felt that Alan was very aware in the afternoon of the release which was coming from his suffering. They were interested to see that he took a few sips of his bourbon before finally going off. "He was so calm,"

---

8. "Probable lethal dose of morphine lies between 120 and 250 milligrams (mg.)—two (2) to four (4) grains. In nonaddicts, therapeutic doses may be dangerously potentiated by alcohol or barbituates. In acute morphinism, death occurs typically within six to twelve hours, nearly always due to respiratory failure." *Clinical Toxology of Commercial Products,* Section III, p. 238. This note refers to morphine taken by mouth.

said his elder daughter, Carol. "It was just like he was going off for a nap. I don't believe he suffered at the end at all. For him it was a dignified death. The heavy breathing and the noise—like snoring—weren't pleasant to us, but I think it was because we weren't used to it."

The funeral home staff came to the Thomas's house at their request within minutes of Alan's death. On arrival the director first telephoned the family physician and asked whether he would sign the death certificate the following day. He was willing. The body was removed immediately to the funeral home, and a few days later Alan Thomas's remains were cremated.

Looking back, nine months later, on the manner of her husband's death, Ruth says: "I should have learned more about drugs and found something which would have killed him more quickly. I am thinking more of myself than I am of him. I don't think he suffered, but it was a long, terrible night for us. I wrongly assumed that the morphine would work faster."

Dr. Browning, a lapsed Catholic who believes in a deity, says, "I knew that Alan was dying, but I didn't know that I was going to be asked to help. It was a Sunday. Had I known in advance, I would have obtained a ten (10) c.c. syringe and a more powerful solution of morphine. I could have given him a lethal dose in one or two injections. I am now better prepared should this ever happen again. Also, I wish I had made better final communication with Alan. That wink helped, but it was not enough. Mentally, I am much better prepared today.

"I have not the slightest regret. I knew all along that this was what should be done. I was convinced of this. When I had to tell my wife later what I had done for Alan, I was wondering about her reaction. But she said, 'You did absolutely right.'"

Asked how he felt about breaking the law in helping Alan to die, Dr. Browning answered, "It doesn't bother me at all. I didn't break any law except that which is written on a piece of paper. As far as I'm concerned I didn't break any moral law, or any God-given law. It didn't and doesn't bother me. I don't believe I broke my Hippocratic oath either. Part of that oath is not to do any harm to people and try to help people. I thought I was not doing harm but good in Alan's case. I thought it was my colleagues who were doing harm in prolonging his pain and suffering. The Hippocratic oath in spirit is what I was doing. It will depend on your interpretation.

"If people choose to call me a murderer I wouldn't like it but I would put up with it, because they are wrong. I don't care to have my true name published because I prefer to make my contribution in a different way. What I want is a change in attitude on voluntary euthanasia because this is something of increasing importance to mankind."

In 1982, Ruth married again.

CHAPTER FOUR

It is silliness to live when to live is torment;
And then have we a prescription to die
When death is our physician.

—WILLIAM SHAKESPEARE

Joan Mercer married an electrician in her home city, Dublin, and had nine children. Years later, when her children were grown and shortly before separating from her husband and moving to England, she developed ovarian cancer which was successfully treated. The method used was called isotope implantation—putting a radioactive capsule inside the body near the cancer to kill the affected cells. (This treatment was widely used in the 1960s but has since been discontinued in favor of other methods with fewer risks.) Not long after she recovered from the cancer, Mrs. Mercer had to have a colostomy (removal of the colon) and was obliged to pass her waste products into a bag for the rest of her life. For many years she was in and out of the hospital with complications.

In the meantime, two of her daughters immigrated to California, one becoming a registered nurse in the northern part of the state, and the other a housewife living near Los Angeles. During the spells when her health was better, Mrs. Mercer loved nothing better than to fly to Los Angeles and spend long holidays with her daughters and their families.

Despite her health problems, Joan Mercer (not her real name) was cheerful and optimistic, denying that she had ever suffered from cancer. Whenever health was being discussed she would insist, "I don't have cancer. I've never had cancer. I don't know what's wrong with me, but it's not cancer."

In 1978 doctors found her kidneys and liver were deteriorating and needed treatment. After being discharged from the hospital, despite the difficulty of travel with a colostomy (particularly in a cramped jet aircraft), Mrs. Mercer returned to California for a holiday. She loved roaming the wild countryside with her daughter and grandson, who were amazed at the mobility and fortitude of the sixty-nine-year old woman. Yet her daughter Margaret detected that underneath all the outward joie de vivre, her mother just might be more deeply depressed than she was letting on, even though Mrs. Mercer vehemently denied this. "I'm definitely not depressed," she would insist. One symptom of low spirits, however, was the fact that she had become a heavy wine drinker, consuming four or five bottles a day.

"What could we do?" recalls Margaret. "The wine picked her up, and she would laugh and giggle. Stella, my sister, is a nurse, and she said that Mother probably did not have long to live anyhow."

Apart from the joy of her holidays in California and the presence of her two daughters there, Mrs. Mercer had a supportive son and daughter living close by in the little village in Somerset, England, where she lived. Yet she preferred keeping them at a distance; she refused to live with them or to let anybody live

26

with her, and she even discouraged the nurses who called to change her tubes from coming too often. If she felt well, she would tell the district nurse, "Go take care of somebody that's sick and leave me alone."

Her abdominal problems worsened, however, and within months she was in and out of the hospital for various treatments. She received a further blow when the son who lived nearby—and had visited her daily—was killed in a car crash only a block from her home when he was on his way to see her. Only twenty-six at the time of his death, he had suffered from leukemia, and his sisters suspected that his death was directly or indirectly a suicide: the fault for the crash was definitely his. They did not communicate this to their mother, but from the depth of her grieving they suspected that she guessed the real reason for his death too.

After her son's death, Mrs. Mercer wept a great deal, drank even more heavily, and made several emotional phone calls to her daughters in California. Realizing that their mother was close to the end, they flew back to England where Mrs. Mercer's doctors confirmed the fact that her health was diminishing and told them she could last anywhere from two weeks to six months.

"She should have been dead ten years ago," commented one physician.

Their mother was indeed in a very bleak state, mentally and physically. Her mouth had festered so badly that she could not eat and could barely drink. She told her daughters, "I have gangrene."

They were able to substantiate with the physician that their mother had "internal gangrene," but Joan Mercer was so upset at the diagnosis that they chose to deny to her that the condition existed. Yet the following day Mrs. Mercer maintained that she knew what she was suffering from: "No, I know I do have gangrene," she said. "I just know I do. I've got to get out now."

Margaret asked her mother what she meant by "getting out." "You know what I mean," she answered. "When I worked in a hospital they had one pill that you give old people to die. They used to give it to them. It's called euthanasia."

Mrs. Mercer surprised her daughters by telling them that she had stolen one of the pills from the hospital.

"Well, where is it?" Stella asked.

"I've put it away somewhere and lost it," wailed their mother. "Is there any way you can get another one for me?"

Both daughters replied that they had no idea where to start looking. They were, after all, no longer accustomed to living in England. They discussed whether one of them could go to London and try to buy some illicit drugs on the street, not an uncommon practice for people desperate to help someone die who have no recourse to a willing and sympathetic physician. Stella recalled that her mother had taken Nembutal[9] for many years, but Mrs. Mercer said that she had exhausted

---

9. If Mrs. Mercer had had a supply of Nembutal (pentobarbital), the minimum lethal dose, according to *The Prediction of Suicide* toxicity chart, is one gram (1 gm.). *The Clinical Toxicology of Commercial Products* (Section II, p. 218) states: "Fatal dose: more than two grams (2 gm.)."

her supply some time previously and could not get any more. Margaret and Stella became frantic as their mother's preoccupation with her gangrene and deterioration intensified. Mrs. Mercer kept referring to it, saying that she knew from her hospital experience that her body would turn black but her mind would remain lucid.

"I can't take any more of this," she said. "I'm totally weak. I'm terribly sick."

The two daughters now devoted all their time to their mother although she was not always a compliant patient, often jumping out of bed when their back was turned and going to the laundryroom where she would start washing clothes. On one occasion Margaret got her mother back to bed and as soon as she had tucked her in Mrs. Mercer said, "You, know, I have prayed to God that He would send one of my children to help me."

"We'll help," said Margaret, aware that her mother meant assistance in helping her to die well.

"I knew you would. I knew you would help me."

Margaret told her mother that she would help her die, but she also wanted time to think about it. "I think we'd better talk about it again," she said. "I don't want to make this decision at this moment. It would be better to talk to you when you have taken no pills. Nothing. I want to be clear that this is not an emotional decision you're making, or that you are depressed."

"No, there is nothing they can do for me now," said Mrs. Mercer. "There's nothing. They will put me in that little hospital in town, and that's where people go to die. They never come out."

Stella added, "Well, maybe you should go into the hospital for one time only and let them check you over and see if there's anything that can be done. Maybe you can be fixed up enough to come back to the States with us and see if we could do anything better back there."

Their mother remained adamant. "I'm not going in the hospital," she declared. "I'll never forgive either one of you if you betray me now, and if you force me into that hospital. That will close off any channels I have of getting out of it."

After a long and thoughtful discussion, the two daughters agreed that it was only right to find some way to help their mother to die. She was, after all, gravely ill. Stella decided to use her status as a nurse to try to get a barbiturate from Mrs. Mercer's physician.

"My mother's not sleeping. She must have a strong sleeping pill" she told him a few days later. "What you have given her is not doing any good."

The doctor prescribed fifty Soneryl, a butabarbital,[10] which in low dosage relieves mild anxiety and in higher dosage induces sleep.

Stella entirely agreed with her mother's decision to end her life, but she did

---

10. In the U.S.A., butabarbital has been sold on prescription since 1939. It has fourteen different brand names, but the best known is Butisol.

not feel able to participate in the act other than getting the sleeping pills from the doctor. It was agreed between the two women that Margaret would administer the actual lethal dose. It was undoubtedly Stella's training as a nurse and the ethics taught her in the hospitals about the importance of saving lives that made her stop short of actively assisting in the death.

The following evening Margaret and Stella noticed that their mother was reviewing her life, talking about her father, her husband, and a multitude of family affairs. She also appeared to be hallucinating.

"My father has been here to see me," she told Margaret. "He stands by the door at night."

"Your father is dead," said Margaret. "Do you know what your are saying?"

"Yes, I know, but I'm not stupid," replied Mrs. Mercer. "I'm telling you he was right here at the door last night. He told me I must come before my next birthday."

Mrs. Mercer was taking Brompton Cocktail (alcohol, cocaine, morphine and a phenathiazine) for pain which, despite the medication, was intensifying. Margaret gave her mother an extra large dose that night to control the increased pain and ensure a good sleep. When she awoke the next morning, Mrs. Mercer commented, "That was the most wonderful sleep I've had in years. I wasn't depressed, and I wasn't lonely."

"I'm glad," Margaret answered.

"Will I sleep like that all the time? Will I never be lonely again?"

"You will never be lonely again," Margaret said. Both she and her sister were relieved that the decision had been made to help their mother die gracefully.

"That's because you and Stella are here." Mrs. Mercer seemed to understand that her daughters were now willing to help her.

The next night Margaret and Stella again gave their mother a strong dose of Brompton Cocktail, and the first thing she said on awakening was, "I had another wonderful night, but I notice that I'm still here."

"Well, what do you think I am, Mother, a hit man from New York?" Stella joked. Both mother and daughter laughed. In fact, throughout the rest of the day there was a lot of bantering between the three women, some of which good-naturedly acknowledged the purpose of their visit.

"What's the use of having all these servants around if I can't get any service?" Mrs. Mercer would tease. The daughters remember it as a happy day, although towards the end of the afternoon the pain and discomfort began to trouble Mrs. Mercer.

"Maggie, I don't want to keep on waking up like this," she said.

"Do you really want out?"

"Yeah, I really want out," said Mrs. Mercer, mimicking her daughter's American accent.

Margaret prodded her mother to try to get at her real feelings, to tell her why she wanted help to die. She still wanted to be absolutely sure of her mother's wishes. "What exactly do you mean, Mother?" she asked.

"I can't go on," was the reply. "What I'm facing, I can't face any more. I can't face the gangrene and the hopelessness of not being able to take care of myself. I really want to go, and I need you to help me do this."

"Do you realize what you are talking about?" Margaret said, quite sharply. She wanted her mother to elucidate clearly exactly what her motives were in wanting to die.

"Absolutely. I realize what I'm talking about. If you don't help me I'll throw myself in the river, or I'll put a plastic bag over my head. There are ways...but I don't know if I could do that. Or if it will work. Can't you get the pills? Can't you get something?"

"Mother, we have," was the final reply. Mrs. Mercer had repeated too many times her desire to die; there was little reason to doubt her now.

There was a pause in the conversation as both women reflected on the seriousness of the decision they were taking.

"It's O.K.," Margaret said. "Stella and I will work on it."

"That would be great."

But Margaret still wanted to be very clear about what was going to happen. There were some niggling worries about the depressing things her mother had been saying about her brother's accident, her bad marriage, and other family troubles, and she wondered if her depression was more emotional that physical. It also bothered her that her mother's final days would be filled with bleak and sad thoughts.

"Now, Mother," she told her. "It's important that if we do this that you have a good frame of mind and don't go out thinking those kinds of thoughts. What I want you to see is a lake, a beautiful lake with white swans and cygnets on it. Everytime you get into Tommy's death or any other stuff, I want you to switch back to the lake with the swans."

Mrs. Mercer could not resist teasing. "You know cygnets are not white when they're born; they're brown."

"Yes I know that, Mother, but sit on the bank with me and watch the swans. Keep pleasant thoughts in your mind and switch off that other stuff every time it comes to your mind. Don't grieve about it anymore. There is nothing that can be done about it. Just keep thinking about the beautiful lake."

Margaret was attempting to give her mother the spiritual comfort she needed during these hours while Stella continued with the nursing and household chores. The two women were an excellent team and good foils for one another. Mrs. Mercer jokingly called Stella the "scullery maid"—the bottom of the English domestic worker scale.

During their vigil they fed their mother baby food, warm broth, and little bits of bread and butter. It was, however, extremely difficult: her mouth was swollen, her tongue seemed to be disintegrating, and there was an alarming swelling on the side of her neck.

Two physicians continued to make regular housecalls. At one point Mrs. Mercer asked one of them, "Would you take me into the hospital and open me up?'' (By this she apparently meant being up on an operating table and allowed to die.) The physician answered that he would not, and afterwards told Margaret that if her mother was operated upon for any reason while in this condition, the subsequent pain would be greater than any amount of heroin could control. ''I would recommend that she never go through another surgery for any reason,'' he commented. ''She has a very large tumor.''

On the sixth day of their vigil Margaret gave Mrs. Mercer some prescribed painkillers mixed in broth to inhibit the pills' bitter taste; at six in the evening, after the broth, her mother asked for some brandy, a normal request at that time of day. Both Margaret and Stella noticed that their mother appeared quite happy and had an anticipatory air about her.

After a pause Margaret finally asked, ''Do you want to take your pills tonight, Mum?''

''Yes, '' was the immediate reply. Margaret noted the lack of hesitation on her mother's part. She left the room and ground up fifteen Soneryl[11] and emptied the powder into a glass containing the usual dose of Brompton Cocktail. As each tablet was 100 milligrams (mg.), this was a dosage of one and a half grams (1.5 gm.).

After returning to the bedroom, Margaret said to her mother, ''This is the medicine, Mom. Do you want to take it?''

There was still a reluctance on the part of both women to use phrases like, ''This will kill you,'' or, ''You won't live after drinking this.'' There was instead an implied understanding about the lethality of the mixture. Mrs. Mercer did not hesitate; without answering she gulped down the liquid, the mixture of Soneryl and Brompton Cocktail. Then Margaret gave her two more pills, her nightly sleeping draught.

''Somehow I wanted to leave her that little bit of comfort that she really did not know what she was taking, when in fact she did,'' she said later on. ''She liked not to completely know, and yet know, too, at the same time.''

After their mother had swallowed the overdose, both Margaret and Stella sat at her bedside, each holding one of her hands. Margaret sang the ballad, ''I'll see you again.''

Before lapsing into sleep Mrs. Mercer whispered, ''God bless you. Thank you so much.''

To stop themselves from crying, the two daughters said the Lord's Prayer and then recited the twenty-third psalm. Mrs. Mercer's last words were, ''Be sure I have a pretty nightgown on when the nurse comes, and don't forget to take the rose to Bill.'' (This was a reference to a painting of a rose which she had done in her youth. She wanted it to go to one of her sons.)

---

11. *The Prediction of Suicide* gives the minimum lethal dose as one gram (1 gm.) in their toxicity chart. *Clinical Toxicology* rates butabarbital sodium as ''extremely toxic.'' Section II, p. 217.

"I will, Mother. I will take it," Margaret assured her.

"Don't forget," Mrs. Mercer replied, and drifted off to sleep.

Stella decided to continue the deathwatch while Margaret retired to rest. They both expected their mother to die in the night but discovered to their dismay that in the morning she was still breathing. She continued to sleep all through Saturday, and when the district nurse called, Margaret suggested that their Mother might have taken too many of her sleeping pills. Perhaps it would be better not to disturb her.

"Oh, I shouldn't think you'd want to do that," said the nurse. "Leave her alone."

Yet the suspense of not knowing whether the overdose would be effective (they had assumed that their mother would be dead within hours of taking the pills) was highly unnerving. What if it failed?

Margaret, agitated and frightened, telephoned the doctor to ask whether her mother could be in pain. "If she's in a very deep sleep, probably a coma, she's not feeling any pain," he said.

"Can you give her a shot?"

"No, I can't. Do you want her to go into the hospital?"

"Oh, no. Not at all."

"I think that's wise," he went on. "Because if she did, they'd pump her stomach and she'd go through all of this again some other time."

His words indicated to Margaret that he had guessed what really happened. "They've been known to come out of a sleep like that after forty-eight hours and be in the same condition as before," he added, a comment which only increased Margaret's and Stella's anxiety.

By now Mrs. Mercer was breathing heavily, which particularly unsettled Margaret. Stella, more accustomed to the situation, tended her mother, clearing mucous from her mouth and checking her bags, which remained empty.

When death had still not come twenty-four hours after administering the overdose, Margaret called the doctor again. He warned her: "It is a terribly distressing thing. Death isn't like it is in the movies. It doesn't happen quickly. It's a slow and sometimes painful process."[12]

Margaret had a sinking feeling that she and her sister had failed. The overdose had not been sufficiently lethal. Their worst fear was that their mother might recover consciousness, but that her brain would be damaged. She and Stella agreed that they should have administered the entire fifty tablets.

Yet after another night, which seemed an eternity and during which time Margaret and Stella steeled themselves for bleak repercussions of their failed attempt, their prayers were finally answered. Joan Mercer stopped breathing just before nine o'clock on Sunday morning.

---

12. James Long states in *The Essential Guide to Prescription Drugs* (p. 88) that the effects of an overdose of butabarbital are "deepening sleep, coma, slow and shallow breathing, weak and rapid pulse, (and) cold and sweaty skin."

Without any questions, two doctors signed the death certificate so that Mrs. Mercer could be cremated. She had given orders that her ashes should be returned to California. "Put them in the flower bed," she had said, "and I'll grow flowers for you."

Margaret recalled later: "Had we known mother was definitely going to die without awakening, it would have been much more bearable for Stella and me. We were terrified that we might have hurt her. Stella never left her side during that coma. She talked to her constantly, saying loving things, just in case she could hear. Had I known Mother was going to ask us to help her die, I would have done some research on drug dosages before I went to England. It was just out of the blue. It was for Stella also, and she is a nurse who is married to a doctor. Given warning, we could have made better preparations."

CHAPTER FIVE

Necessity hath no law.

—OLIVER CROMWELL.

The Hemlock Society does not, of course, approve of mercy killing. The quintessence of voluntary euthanasia is personal choice and self-control, with sometimes a little help from one's friends. Mercy killing, on the other hand, is the unrequested taking of one person's life by another in order to save that person further suffering. The death is often unasked for because the patient is unable to communicate his or her wishes. Mercy killing is an act of incredible desperation, and frequently the life-taker is suffering from, or is near to, an emotional collapse because of strain of caring for someone terminally ill. Witnessing the endless suffering of a loved one with no sign of imminent release has become unendurable. Pushed to intolerable limits, the individual feels compelled to hasten death—by whatever means—because no one else will.

Mercy killers are usually confronted with a criminal charge of murder or manslaughter. Up until twenty years ago in Western society an act of mercy killing between husband and wife or parent and child, committed for the most compassionate reasons, often brought a death sentence, later commuted to life imprisonment. Since then, the sentences have diminished as judges recognize the merciful nature of the "crime." In more recent years the punishment is frequently probation with the stipulation that the defendant undergo psychiatric treatment. In the USA in recent years there have been cases where juries have refused to indict or convict 'mercy killers,' even against the weight of evidence.

When the goals of the voluntary euthanasia movement are achieved, mercy killing will virtually cease to exist as a crime. More importantly, it will put an end to the additional and needless human suffering.

We report the following case of a mercy killing, not to condone or condemn the actions of any of the individuals, but to help all of us better understand the complexity of decision-making in the process of dying, as well as the medical and legal obstacles inherent in such a situation. Most of all, the story tells us of the misjudgements made by individuals reduced to such desperate action because they had no one to guide or counsel them.

Frank Robinson (his real name) never hesitates to point out that he and his mother enjoyed lots of love, both in his childhood and as a grown man. "Mom played a great deal with us kids," he says. "We grew up very close." Frank has often been derided by colleagues as a "mother's boy" because, after twenty years apart, he and his mother set up home together once again. He answers such derision thus: "I always say, if you live with your father they never say you're a father's boy. I'm not the marrying type. She was my friend. My buddy. She was easy-going, good-natured, I could talk to her. We had similar natures."

Frank was born in Patterson, New Jersey, in 1925, the son of a policeman of English-Irish extraction. His mother, Irene, was of Dutch ancestry. There was another child, a daughter, Anna. The marriage did not last long, and after the divorce his mother worked long hours in laundries or restaurants during the Depression to bring up her children.

As a Christian believer she brought up her family to read the Bible every Sunday although she did not attach herself to any religious denomination. Instead she seemed to have her own religion founded on a simple faith in God. Frank had been baptized a Roman Catholic because of his father's beliefs, but after the dissolution of the marriage he dropped Catholicism and followed his mother's more homespun theology.

At fifteen Frank moved to Cincinnati, Ohio, with his mother and the man she was then living with. He became a water boy and cement finisher's apprentice, and at seventeen he enlisted in the Marine Corps, serving as an anti-aircraft gunner fighting the Japanese in Midway and Okinawa in the final stages of the Pacific conflict.

When peace came he took several jobs in New Jersey before settling down to employment for twelve years as a power linesman. Then, after a series of accidents, he quit and in 1959 he re-enlisted in the Marines. For the next four years he served in the Cuban blockade and did two tours of duty in the Mediterranean. During this time his sister died when she was thirty-eight of cancer, and his mother was briefly married to a man named Harris. When Frank came out of the service he and his mother, now aged 60, decided to start a new life together in California.

Thirteen years later, after a series of incidents when she had passed out for no apparent reason, it was discovered that Irene Harris was diabetic. She gave up odd jobs she was doing, and Frank willingly supported the two of them. Unfortunately, his mother developed high blood pressure as well, and on two occasions Frank came home from work to find that she had been rushed to the hospital after a collapse. To add to her ailments, she also suffered from severe arthritis of the knees.

"She was starting to deteriorate to the point where the quality of her life really changed," recalls Frank. Although only five feet three inches tall, Irene weighed well over two hundred pounds. Because of the complexity of the health problems and her heaviness, she had great difficulty travelling very far and consequently rarely left the apartment in West Los Angeles where she and Frank lived.

Doctors warned Mrs. Harris and her son that she was a candidate for a serious stroke because of her high blood pressure. When she learned this, Irene told Frank, "If I should start to go, don't try to save me. And don't put me in a convalescent home. That's a place of the living dead."

Irene knew that because Frank loved her, he would undoubtedly struggle to keep her alive as long as possible. This was her first attempt to clarify her wishes. Frank was embarrassed by her request not to save her but agreed that he would not admit her to a convalescent home. He remarked rather flippantly, "Don't worry, Mom, I'll shoot you first."

His mother laughed. "You couldn't hurt a fly," she added.

On September 14, 1979, Irene went to the laundry room in her apartment complex and there suffered a massive stroke. The apartment managers could not locate Frank at his office and when he reached home at six p.m. that evening, he learned that she was at St. John's Hospital in Santa Monica. After rushing there, he was informed that his mother was completely paralyzed on her right side and could neither speak nor eat. She was in the Intensive Care Unit.

A week later she was listed as medically "stable" and moved from intensive care to a ward. After another week, a doctor telephoned Frank at work and told him, "I believe it's hopeless. Your mother will never again talk or walk. It seems a cruel thing to say. But then again, in time it may change."

That evening, after the telephone call, Frank went to the hospital as usual. Suddenly his mother began to twist and turn strangely while he sat beside her. Alarmed, he called a nurse who in turn called a doctor.

The doctor took one look and said, "It's another stroke. She's going fast. Maybe it's better to let her go."

Although it was contrary to what he had promised his mother, Frank was so upset at seeing her so close to death that he said, impulsively, "Can't you help her?"

"Do you want a lot of expensive machinery?" the doctor asked. "Is her quality of life that good?"

"No, let her go," Frank said, but almost immediately he started to weep as he recalled that his mother had not been entirely disabled before the latest stroke. "But she was able to go to the store," he cried feebly. Looking back on that crucial moment at the hospital, Frank admits that he was too distraught by the thought of losing his mother to think clearly. He forgot about her request to let her die. It was a moment he would deeply regret.

"Oh, she was, was she?" replied the doctor, nodding to the nurse who then injected Irene with a stimulant for the heart.

"Help, her, doctor," Frank cried.

In spite of the injection, Irene was not expected to last through the night. Frank returned home, frightened and bewildered, thinking that he had lost his mother. When he telephoned the hospital the next day, however, he was told that his mother's condition had "stabilized," although she was still in a desperate physical condition. On his evening visit Frank found her the same: paralyzed, unable to speak and being fed through a tube in her nose.

He sat quietly, observing his mother and pondering the events of the previous evening. Why had he cried out to keep her alive? The crucial events in the ward had all happened in what seemed like less than a minute. He blamed himself in part for his inability to let his mother die, but he also felt that the doctor had been wrong in bombarding him with so many questions at such a stressful time. He had been in a muddle because of the emotional strain of seeing the only person he loved in the world leaving him. Would she have lived anyway? There were so many unknowns.

For the next sixty-five days Irene Harris lay in the hospital, being turned ever two hours to prevent bedsores and being fed by the tube which she constantly tried to pull out of her nose with her one useful hand. She received excellent care from the staff of St. John's and in return she tried to be a good patient. When a nurse had finished tending her she would clutch at her hand and kiss it. The nurses took the trouble to braid her hair and on any special occasion they would entwine flowers with the braids.

By the end of this time a hospital social worker began to put pressure on Frank to take his mother out of St. John's, which is specifically for the care of the acutely sick and injured, and urged him to put her into a nursing home for the aged and infirm. He agreed to consider it. After looking at several nursing homes, however, he came to a single conclusion: "They're pigsties. The first thing which hit me was that they were old buildings, they stank of urine, the rooms were shabby-looking, and the general appearance of the premises and grounds were decrepit. The attitude of the people was bad. Such things as call lights were ignored."

The social worker at St. John's did her best to guide Frank towards the most suitable homes and, when he failed to find anything—either because the homes were too full or too disgusting for him to tolerate—she admitted, "Let's face it, nobody wants her. She's too heavy. They prefer the little skinny, eighty-pounders. And she can't go to the bathroom to relieve herself. She needs too much nursing."

The hospital subsequently tried to arrange nurses to take care of Irene at home, and Frank was able to secure a hospital bed and have it installed in his apartment. (Medicare paid for this.) Three days before she was due to return home, however, the apartment was burgled, and about $350—which was for the nurse's fees—their television, radio, and many personal effects were all stolen. This was the last straw. The combined effects of visiting his mother every night and preparing for her homecoming, compounded by the shock of the burglary, began to affect Frank's health. For several weeks he had been unable to sleep more than a few minutes at a time, and he now found himself unable to swallow solid food. He began to be haunted by a fear that if his mother came home, he would be forced to take her life, not only for her sake, but because he realized that he was close to a breakdown. After a doctor told him that his mother could continue to live anywhere from one to ten years longer, he did not trust his self-control.

"My first thought of hearing this was that I would take my mother's life," he said later. "That I wouldn't let her go through that. I thought of shooting her. I had a small twenty-two caliber Deringer which I had bought for my own

37

protection years before when I lived in a dangerous neighborhood. Not a very lethal gun except if you hit the person in the right place. I knew what she had been going through in recent months. I loved my mother so much that I could feel what she felt. I was taking afternoons off from work and visiting her twice a day. There was a reason for this: I went in one evening and, as good as the nursing was, I saw my mother had a pained look on her face. The nurse had rolled my mother on her paralyzed arm. She couldn't reach her call bell. Another time I saw a demented woman frightening my mother. When I saw things like that, how could I stay away?"

"I remember thinking that my mother's not going to live as a vegetable. I said to myself, 'I'll blow her away.' I was angry, not at my mother, but angry that this should happen to me. Why me? I asked a priest why, and he said to ask God. I didn't want to shoot her. I told doctors not to keep her alive. I would chase them out of the room when they used that machine to push fluid down her lungs. She told me she didn't want that. I wanted her to go with God. God takes you in His way, but the doctors were fighting against nature, so how could she go? I knew what the end result was going to be: bedridden, with bedsores.

"So I started asking people about medication which would take my mother's life. But no one would tell me. A L.V.N. (partly qualified nurse) who lives in these apartments said a triple shot of insulin would do it. I asked my niece who is an R.N. back in New Jersey, and she said she would call back and then she never did. I asked my mother's own physician to put her to sleep and he said he would see what he could do and call back. He didn't either. And he had been her physician for seventeen years."

By the time Frank realized that no one was going to help him, he was in such a chaotic state of mind that he could not organize himself enough to find out any further information on lethal drug overdoses. Now obsessed with the thought that he had to keep his promise to his mother and help her end her life, he lacked the mental resources to research the subject properly.

Further pressure came from the hospital. They now advised him that if he did not remove his mother immediately, they would be obliged to charge him $200 a day for her care. Up to that point, Medicare had been paying all the bills.

Rather hastily, on November 17, Frank put his mother in a nearby convalescent home, one not at all to his liking. It had the same pervading smell of urine, and although it looked fairly decent from the outside, Frank saw cockroaches in the rooms. On several visits he found his mother's bell-call apparatus lying on the floor and attendants watching the patients' television (for which he was paying rental). He also found that his mother would be kept up in a chair for two hours, whereas St. John's had only kept her up for fifteen minutes. When he complained that this tired and pained her, the staff replied that they had the right to keep her in a chair for as long as they wished.

In the meantime, Irene was gaining even more weight—she was now well over two hundred and thirty pounds—which made it extremely difficult for the nurses or attendants to turn her over. One day Frank went into the home and found her face was covered with hardened matter which he feared was excrement. He got a washcloth to clean it off and found that it was caked food. It turned out that Irene, forced to feed herself, had been using her one hand to thrust food in her mouth and was so clumsy that she spattered most of it over her face.

Disgusted and angry at the appalling care his mother was getting, he decided to complain. Nobody was taking the trouble to feed her or even look after her hygiene in the most fundamental ways. Yet when he vented his anger, he was told by the staff, "Don't complain, Mr. Robinson, or we'll ask you to take her out of here."

Irene was supposed to be turned every two hours to prevent bed sores, but for a month Frank never saw any evidence that this was being done. His mother was supposed to eat only soft food; one day he found her eating a large hamburger and he was afraid she would choke. For once his complaint was heeded and her diet was changed. On balance, however, he was alarmed at the staff's neglect, and on December 17 he decided to try looking after his mother at home. Despite the fact that Medicaid had paid for almost all of the expenses in the nursing home, he though that it would be nice for them to be together during the Christmas holidays.

Yet after only twenty-four hours at home, a visiting nurse discovered that Irene had an infection in her catheter. There was also a blockage in her stomach and her bowels were like a drum. She was rushed to St. John's Hospital again, where she stayed for three weeks to clear up these problems. She was now on a double catheter to drain her bowels and her bladder.

It was during that spell in the hospital, Frank recalls, that his mother asked him to shoot her.

"When I say 'asked'," he points out, "it was kind of indirect. Because she couldn't talk, she took her left hand, with her thumb held up vertically and the forefinger extended horizontally in the shape of a gun, and she put her hand to her temple in a mock suicide. I pulled a dummy act, like, 'I don't know what you mean, Mom.' Then she did it again. I said to her, 'Mom, do you want me to take your life?' and she nodded. I told her that it would be best not to let it happen here because somebody else might get hurt. I told her to wait until I got her home."

In the weeks before his mother was discharged from the hospital Frank told several acquaintances that if he did not get some help he would take his mother's life. Their response was invariably noncommittal. "Oh, don't think like that," they would say, or, "You shouldn't do that." Some walked away. Nobody offered any real advice or comfort, and certainly no one offered any help. Frank approached an attorney in his apartment complex whom he knew and pointedly asked what would happen if he shot his mother. The attorney ducked the question by saying that as he was not a criminal lawyer he did not know the answer. "You should ask someone more qualified," he commented dryly. The family doctor was approached once again about helping Irene to die.

"Don't talk to me like that," replied the doctor. "I'm not going to do it."

"O.K.," Frank said. "Then I'll do it myself. I'm breaking down. I'm falling apart."

It is incontrovertible that Frank warned society about what he intended to do to his mother. No one helped him.

Frank's mental and physical health continued to deteriorate. The strain of visiting his mother twice a day, sitting for hours beside her bed with her unable to communicate, combined with the worry of what was going to happen, all contributed to his decline. There was no other family member in California or even a close friend who could help with the burden. Because of his increased isolation, Frank had no moral support from anyone. Although he was a pleasant, gregarious man, and was well-liked in the community for his participation in sports events, he discovered that people would make vague sympathetic noises about his mother's condition but never actually volunteer to do anything or even to visit her.

"The worst thing of all was when I came home from the hospital and I was all alone, with no one to hold onto," recalls Frank. "I was going mad. Then I started hearing voices. Not voices from you to me, but inside my head. I became two people. The voices would say, 'Don't go to the hospital. You'll be sorry.' I would get in my car and hear a voice. 'There's going to be trouble,' it would say."

During his visits Irene now began to make guttural sounds which upset him. He tried to convince himself that she was singing. When he could no longer bear the sight and sounds of her distressing condition he would go to the end of the corridor for a cigarette where he could still hear her cries. "Don't pay any attention to it," the nursing staff would say.

In his desperate state, Frank frequently asked the doctors and nurses to give his mother "something to put her to sleep," meaning, of course, to end her life. When Irene again made the simulated shooting motions with her hand, and the meaning of the gesture was unmistakable, Frank was so overcome that he grasped his mother in his arms to kiss her and was surprised that she, too, grabbed him tightly. She would not let go.

"I think she thought I was going to shoot her then," says Frank. "My mother wanted that."

He had by then lost forty pounds, had badly strained, bloodshot eyes from lack of sleep and looked worn out. He could tell from his mother's eyes that she was worried about the way he was affected by her illness.

After some deliberation he took his gun to the hospital one night with the intention of shooting his mother. Her message to him had been clear; he felt that it was now time to act. Fortifying himself with several drinks beforehand, he was careful not to have so much that the security guards and nursing staff at the hospital would notice that he was inebriated. Throughout the preparations he was aware that if he tried to shoot Irene and failed he would be imprisoned. That would be letting his mother down. She would then have no one in the world, and it would be the same as abandoning her. Reaching her hospital room, he showed his mother the gun and indicated that he wanted her to take it and kill herself, if she chose. Then he quickly changed his mind.

"I didn't want to shoot my mother, and when she took the gun and waved it around, I was terrified that she would shoot the woman in the next bed. I took it away from her quickly, and told her to wait until we got home. That seemed to pacify her." But his plan had failed.

By then it was the week of Christmas and Frank returned to his apartment that evening to sit and meditate, listening to the carols floating through his window and the sound of other people's parties. He became morbidly depressed, knowing how much he and his mother were suffering while others were so happy. His failure to carry out his plan of shooting his mother—or her shooting herself—deepened his depression.

Early in the new year of 1980, Frank removed his mother once again from St. John's because the hospital said that if he did not, they would be obliged to put her in an institution on the grounds that she was considered "abandoned." The institution might be up to fifty miles away, and he would not be able to visit her. Once again he brought his mother home, except that now he arranged to pay a woman from a nursing agency fifty dollars to stay with his mother during the day. That first day Frank did the "evening watch." As he sat beside his mother he was at once overwhelmed by the immensity of the problems facing him. Whenever he turned on the television his mother twisted and turned and groaned until it was switched off. Frank wondered how he could exist sitting beside her every evening for an indefinite period of time without any escape or distraction. In that silent room he pondered how long his money would last. There were still some savings but he estimated that it was going to average seven hundred dollars a week to care for Irene. In about two months the savings would be depleted.

Before he went to bed that night his mother seemed to be fairly conscious of what was going on so Frank talked to her. He explained why he had not brought her home before, asking her forgiveness. He talked about the intense strain on himself. Irene appeared to understand and responded with her eyes which seemed to be alert and understanding.

Frank told her, "Mom, believe me, I love you, but there's only one answer. But if I take your life, I will go to prison. Do you want me to go to prison?"

Irene nodded. Frank asked her the same question a second time. Again Irene nodded. Frank left the room, lit a cigarette and sat on his bed, trying to think things through.

"I realized that if she could go through the torture of being in bed twenty-four hours a day, unable to speak, with all those tubes connected to her, then I could do the other," Frank remembers. "I opened up the drawer with the gun, and I heard as clear as day the voice say, 'Frank, take the gun and shoot your mother.' (I've been asked since whose voice this was, God or the Devil, but I don't know.) I felt calm, like I was in a play. I took the gun, I walked out, and I put it on the back of my mother's head. My hands started shaking. I couldn't do it if she was sleeping. She was too peaceful. She looked too nice to me. It had to be when she was making that funny noise. I went back into my bedroom and waited. I tried to get some sleep. It got to about four in the morning, and I walked out again. She made this horrible noise, and the gun went off. I was surprised. I had shot my mother in the back of the head. I thought, 'My God! I've done it!' And I went in my bedroom and then heard another gurgling sound and my first thought was, 'I'm butchering my mother! She's not dead'.''

"And I walked out and I shot my mother again in the head. I went back in the bedroom thinking that that had done it when I heard a moan. My intention had been to take my mother's life quickly, and I was afraid. I ran out and put the gun to her chest and fired again. I felt the life go out of my mother. I felt the relief come off my shoulders like the world had come off. After that, I don't know what I did. I made a cup of coffee and sat on my bed. Then fear came. I thought they were going to put me in prison for a very long time.

"I looked at my dead mother and I kissed her and said, 'Go to God.' I pulled the sheet over her head and put a figurine of the Madonna on her chest.''

In his panic-stricken state Frank decided to draw all his money out of the bank and run. But as he was leaving with his bag packed with clothes he noticed that a neighbor saw him. Tossing the suitcase into a trash can he then got into his car. He drove around West Los Angeles aimlessly, nearly knocking down several pedestrians, but he still had the presence of mind to post a letter to the Neptune Society telling them to cremate his mother.

At about eight a.m. Frank found himself driving past the Veterans' Administration Hospital in Westwood. Here he realized might be sanctuary. He had visited there some weeks before, informing them that he feared he would shoot his mother. They had prescribed Valium. He parked his car and went inside to see a psychiatric worker.

"This is an emergency," he said. "I've just taken my mother's life. Call the police."

The staff gave him a strong tranquilizer and called the Los Angeles police, who subsequently took him to Venice police station where he remained in custody for five days. Frank spurned their suggestion that he get a lawyer to protect his interests.

"If you shoot me, I don't care," was his response.

Finally, however, he capitulated, and an attorney was contacted who agreed to represent him at an hourly fee of a hundred and twenty five dollars. Frank at that point was indifferent to the size of the fee.

If his acquaintances failed to help him while his mother was ill, at least they did not let him down once he had shot her. A petition was circulated in the apartment complex and signed by nearly three hundred people. In it was the declaration that Frank was known to be a law-abiding person, was a good son and had loved his mother. The petitioners asked the courts to show him mercy.

Another group signed a large decorated card wishing him well.

When he appeared before a judge in Santa Monica Court, Frank's lawyer exhibited these expressions of sympathy in court and as a direct result Frank was bailed on his own recognizance. He agreed to be admitted to the psychiatric ward of the Veterans' Administration Hospital, remaining there for two and a half months. It was a fortunate decision. It became a haven from the troubles of the world, and Frank received excellent medical and psychiatric help. He was quite willing—and relieved—to talk to his counsellors about what he had done because he wanted guidance in understanding his act. He also wanted other people to know what he had experienced.

"I was the sanest person in that ward," says Frank. "I knew I had done something which they considered terrible, but I wasn't afraid to talk about it and come to grips with it."

Frank's lawyer negotiated with a considerate District Attorney who moved the case before a judge who was known to be responsive and sympathetic. The charge was reduced from murder to "assault with a deadly weapon" and Frank pleaded guilty. He received three years' probation with a condition that he remain in the care of the Veterans' Administration.

The judge told Frank, "I think in similar circumstances I would have done the same thing to my mother. But the court cannot condone this."

Frank's legal bills amounted to $4,625. He made only two brief appearances in court, totalling about fifteen minutes. The attorney's primary duties were behind-the-scenes negotiations.

Looking back a year after the shooting, Frank comments: "When you take the life of someone you love, you take your own life. In this past year I've felt dead inside. I sleep but I don't rest. There is something in my subconscious troubling me. I can control it by day, but when I go to sleep that monster starts churning. Even though I did right, if you do something that your brains and your eyes don't approve of, it wants to get out.

"It helps to talk. I had no other choice but to kill my mother unless I wanted to disintegrate to where I went out and became a basket case. It's not guilt I feel, or else I couldn't continue living. It's a terrible act. What more can you ask of a person than that they kill someone they love, or even assist? But that doesn't mean that the head is completely clear. That's why I sleep but do not rest.

"The few people who do feel able to talk to me invariably ask, 'Why the gun?' I ask them what they would have used. Where do you get the drugs with which a person can take their life? If I'd had one of those cyanide pills the Nazis used, I could have said to her, 'Mom, take your pill.' It would have been beautiful. I could have sat and held her hand. But that wasn't an option I had."

"The hardest part is now. Living with what happened. It's taken me a year to get over crying. Every day I've thought of what happened. Every day I've cried. I've thought of suicide. I've had so much anger, I thought of killing my

43

mother's physician. I also thought of buying a shotgun and going down to the nursing home and clearing the place out. Unless you've been in my position you don't know what it's like. There's a whole message I want to give to the world about this but nobody wants to listen. It is that I don't want this to happen to the next person.

"It's my life. I'm in this body and no one, including God, has the right to tell me that I have the right to suffer when it's time to go. Everbody thinks that when they are going to die it's going to be easy. Like in combat, it's the other guy who gets shot. It doesn't work that way. I say, let's take control of it."

CHAPTER SIX

We feel we are greater than we know.

This account of the last hours of an 83-year-old woman in Arizona does not illustrate a good death. We publish it partly to demonstrate how difficult it can be to die well without the practical help of a physician. In this case an assisted suicide was bungled and turned into a mercy killing. Mary McFee (not her real name) decided after a good deal of agonizing that suffocating her mother was essentially an act of compassion, not of brutality, saving the elderly lady from weeks, perhaps months, of needless suffering.

Secondly, Mary's story illustrates the ambivalence most people feel about the "rightness' of helping someone to die. Mary's conscience was further disrupted by the fact that she had been estranged from her mother almost all her life. Up until a few months before her mother's death, the two women despised each other. Then there was a late reconciliation, meaningful and beautiful to both.

When she had to help her mother to die, however, Mary was stricken with remorse about whether she was doing this to get her mother "out of the way" and to save herself the trouble of nursing her. The method by which she gauged the reality of the situation and arrived at her own criteria for deciding is narrated in Mary's own words.

In her girlhood, Mary's mother had led an unhappy life. She was the unwanted child of an older married couple who had not desired any more children, and she was something of a burden to them after rheumatic fever left her slightly deaf. As a young woman, she took up nursing in Virginia and became engaged to a doctor. While they were courting, the fiance was murdered in front of her by a jealous rival. It took several years for her to recover from this shock, but eventually she became engaged to another doctor. This love affair, however, broke off when he became a morphine addict. Eventually she married another man, and the couple moved to Arizona to start their new life together. Mary was born soon afterwards. The marriage, unfortunately, was not a happy one, and her parents were divorced when Mary was five years old. Mary describes her growing up with her mother as "painful to look back upon," and at 16 she left home for good. There were several attempts at reconciliation over the years, but these were invariably fruitless and ended up with bitter arguments, only deepening the estrangement. In her early fifties her mother married again, once more unluckily. Her husband died of bone cancer after only two years of marriage.

Over the next twenty years, there was nominal communication between the two women. For another five years there was virtually no contact until one day, totally unexpectedly, Mary received a cryptic note from her mother. "Please contact me when you receive this," it said. Travelling several hundred miles to the city where her mother lived, Mary found her living in a small apartment complex for senior citizens. It was a warm, comfortable home, but her mother had seriously declined in health, apparently from a series of minor strokes.

Because of her illness, her mother was upset at the prospect of leaving the home she loved and entering a nursing home, explaining that that was why she had contacted her daughter. Mary offered whatever help she could give (which was not a great deal at that time other than moral support) and returned to her home in the northern part of the state. It was not long, however, before there was another cry for help. The old lady telephoned in late November, 1979, to say she was unwell.

"Mom, how can I help you?" Mary asked.

"Well, if you could come and help me find a place," she said. "Or you could just call places on the telephone, that would help."

"I'll do better than that. I'll come down."

Mary planned to fly down on the thirteenth of December, but on the twelfth there was a call to say that her mother had suffered a severe heart attack and had been taken to an intensive care unit at the local hospital. Mary flew south immediately and went to the hospital. Her own account as told to me begins now:

When I walked into the Intensive Care Unit, my mother looked like she was already dead. She just looked really, really bad. And my first emotional response was, "Oh dear, why didn't they let her die?" She was eighty-three and she was so depressed at the prospect of going into a nursing home. And I thought, it's time for her to die; why don't they just let people die when they're supposed to? I sat down and talked to my mother and she was very, very anxious. She had a sense that she was dying, and she was desperate to get out things that she wanted to say. She said that she had been thinking a lot over the last few years. She said that when she thought back, and thought about why people had done the things they'd done, she couldn't be mad at them anymore. I was so proud of her, for a crazy lady.

She included everybody in that. She had never before forgiven anybody. This was one of her things, she never forgave anybody a grudge. And another aspect of her paranoia was that when people would be merely thoughtless, she would read into their thoughtlessness a malicious motive. This was for me perhaps the most painful part of it because as a child you know you are thoughtless, and my mother kept telling me that I was malicious and that I did all these terrible things. So that was a special moment in the hospital, and I thought: Oh, isn't this wonderful that she got that far before she died. And then I began to be glad she hadn't died. Because, I thought, just to hear my mother say that made it worthwhile.

One of the enormous senses I had of my mother's life was of waste. A woman with potential talent, who had a great deal of charm even in her eighties, and who I think was basically extremely intelligent, but who just pissed away her life. Eighty years of nothing, eighty years sitting inside an egg hating everybody, and thinking that everybody wanted to break her eggshell. That's how my mother spent her life. And I was so grateful for just one thing—her words about forgiveness—and I was glad she lasted till I got there. At that time I thought she was bound to go anytime; she really looked bad.

But she didn't get any worse so a doctor said she should go to a retirement home. I couldn't absorb that, but there were lots of things going on for me. One was that I was very ill myself, and I was emotionally devastated by all this stuff and my confidence in my own judgment got clouded. I thought she shouldn't go to a rest home, but I knew the state I was in. At the time I could only think— "I'm awfully emotional and I don't feel well and I just don't trust my own judgment and surely this doctor knows what he's saying. He's reputedly the best cardiologist in the area."

So I didn't fight him on that and I took her to a rest home and left her there and went back up north. Then not long after I got this pitiful phone call one morning about seven-thirty and my mother was crying and she said, "Come and get me." She sounded like a little child. I asked, "What's the matter?" She really couldn't tell me, she wasn't coherent, but by that time I had rested a little bit and I was more in control of myself. I thought, my mother doesn't belong there, she cannot cope. She was in a retirement home which had no nursing care.

I went down south and had my mother flown up to my home and had her admitted to a nursing home. I felt that if there were any more crises like that, I couldn't be flying nine hundred miles once a month. She then appeared to have a series of small strokes. I would go one day and my mother would be alert and I'd go three days later and she would say, "You know, something funny is happening to me. I will start a sentence and then I can't remember the end of the sentence when I get to it." She said, "Do I seem funny to you?"

She was able to walk just a little but she didn't seem to be getting better; she seemed worse. Her mind did seem less alert. It's quite clear that she had a series of small strokes. But she didn't get the typical paralysis on one side of the body so nobody acknowledged that she had had a stroke.

When she went into the nursing home she realized that she had lost the home that she loved, and for the rest of her life she would be dependent. Other people seemed to accept the life all right but my mother did not. She was really depressed. She deteriorated very fast, and she would sometimes look at the other people and she'd say: "Oh, I can't stand it. I can't stand it, if I ever get like that." And she would say that repeatedly. There were some very pitiful cases there. One day she was telling me about a lady down the hall, and she said, "She's just a vegetable , she can't even talk and somebody has to feed her, and when I think that may happen to me..." And then she broke down and started crying.

It just hit me really hard. One of the things that was happening was that something was being awakened in me that I had never felt before: it was a really profound love for my mother. And it was a different kind of love to that which I had felt as a child. I was so proud of her because she wasn't really depressed; she was trying so hard to adjust. And my mother, who had never said a nice thing to me in all her life that I can remember except to impress somebody else, who never gave me credit for performing well at anything, said to me at one point: "You've done everything you can to make me comfortable and to keep me from worrying." And I was so grateful. It was the first praise I had from her. I said, "I've certainly tried, Mother." There were little events like that.

The significance of these events to me was the tremendous growth in her and, you know, that's why I loved her so much, for through all this pain she was at last growing, the first growth I'd seen in her in her entire life. She tried to do the best for me. Sometimes, for instance, it would be apparent that she had been rehearsing before I got there to tell me cheerful, upbeat things so that I would not know how profound her depression was. And I was so touched. In other words, I felt like my mother loved me for the first time.

One day she said that she had seen a number of people like vegetables, and I just knew that I didn't want that to happen to her. For her this was the worst nightmare that could possibly happen. I knew my mother was not the kind of person who would ever be able to take the initiative of suggesting it herself, so when we went back to her room she had to go into the toilet and I had to go help her. She wasn't able to get up from the toilet by herself and I wrote: "Do we need to go back to the bathroom?" She nodded. So we went. I closed the door of the bathroom, but even that way there was no privacy. I scribbled on a piece of paper, "Mother, if you ever become like the woman down the hall, do you want me to give you some pills?" And when she read the note her face just lit up like the sun. She had this look of joy and she looked at me and all she said was, "Oh, you sweet child." And that was the totality of our agreement.

It was not very long after that she got really worse. There was a day when she said to me, "I wonder if this is the beginning of the end?" And I said, "Yes, Mother, I think it is. But I'm going to stay with you all the way." And I reached over and took her arm, which is something that would have been unthinkable before. I never touched my mother before. It was never allowed.

But at that moment she cut off. I though, gee, it would be wonderful if my mother could talk about her death and let me help her in some way, but that was the end for then, and she looked away and withdrew. As in a very typical way, the old way.

The next time I saw her she had gotten out of bed and fallen and broken her hip and she was mad as a hatter. She said she was going on a helicopter ride, and she was obviously delirious. They took her to the hospital from the nursing home. This was another nightmare. God, it was awful. Hours she had been lying there with a broken hip. I was the one who found out. She had fallen out of bed and they put her back, and nobody noticed that she was having all this pain. When I came I said, "Is something wrong with my mother?" I found out from one of the nurses' aids, who I'm sure wasn't supposed to tell me, but she let it slip, that my mother had taken a fall three days before. For three days she had lain there with a broken hip.

At the hospital it was the same, where we sat around for hours with her on a

48

urine-drenched sheet—which they wouldn't let me remove—till they took X-rays because they didn't want to roll her around. I said, "Why does she have to lie on this thing?" It really stank. When they had come to take her to the hospital, my mother understood where she was going, and her remark was, "Oh, what's the use?" She was clear enough to say that. And then when she was in the X-ray room at the hospital, going through all this crap, she finally started to roll her head back and forth and she said, "no more, no more, no more, please no more." Just over and over again. The next time I saw her they had operated on her hip, and she had no mind left at all. sometimes she would act like she was glad to see me, but I was never sure if she knew who I was. I asked her one time if she knew who I was and she said, "Yes, you're William."

All her mental capacity was gone. she was just short of being a vegetable. She could still respond sometimes, but most of the time she was really out of it.

About this time I wrote to a doctor I know and in the letter I said: "You are the only person I feel that I dare ask to help me with this, but would you please help us..." I explained our dilemma. And he called me up and he said, "Yes, I've done the same for a mother of a friend." And he made a recommendation of what to do. It involved a drug that my mother had been taking, called Digoxin, which slows the heartbeat, so if you give an overdose it stimulates a heart attack.[13] But he said under no circumstances should I do it in a hospital. I said, "My God! I don't know how long she'll be there!" He said the overdose should be about four or five times whatever the amount she was taking. So I had to make sure of the amount she was receiving. He repeated under no circumstances should I do it in the hospital, although I felt they were so negligent there that you could probably do anything. He was very concerned about my welfare.

My mother stayed there about ten more days, and then they said she could be released. They wanted her to go to an extended care unit in a nursing home. I said, "There is no way my mother is ever going back to a nursing home; she is coming home with me." So they released her to me, and I took her home. By the time I got her home there was no recognition, ever. And she was just really fading. I knew that she was dying fast, but I had some home health service people come over and I discussed this with them. I said that it seemed to me that my mother was dying. "What do you think?" I asked. "You have experience with terminal patients." Unanimously they said, "Well, it's funny about that. You know, especially with stroke patients, sometimes it will just be clear to everybody that they are going, and then they will live for a year or two years."

---

13. Digoxin, a derivative of the digitalis plant, is rated as "super toxic" by *Clinical Toxicology,* which says that (Section II, p. 165) "an estimated single lethal dose is (between) ten and twenty milligrams (10 and 20 mg.)." Dreisbach states in *Current Medical Diagnosis and Treatment* (edited by Krupp and Chatton; Lange Medical Publications, Los Altos, California, 1981) on p. 961 that "the minimum lethal dose (m.l.d.) of digitalis is three grams (3 gm.) and that of digitoxin three milligrams (3mg.)." Note that toxic doses cause very uncomfortable persistent nausea and vomiting.

They said the sad part of that is it's so hard for the family because they get themselves resigned and ready for it, and then it drags on for ever and ever. And I said, "Oh dear."

In the meantime my mother was in pain. She could not communicate, but from the way her face looked I felt like somewhere she was aware of herself, her pain, and the situation she was in. So I made the decision that I was going to go ahead and do this, to help her.

She was brought home on a Thursday and I gave her her pills on the Saturday morning, very early. I had changed my mind about what I was going to give her. She was getting a pain pill, Phenaphen No. Three, so I looked in the *Physician's Desk Reference* book and in the cautionary notes it was described as a far more lethal medication that Digoxin. The book says that a severe overdose can result in respiratory and cardiac failure, as well as possibly result in acute hepatic toxicity.[14]

I mulled it over and for some reason I didn't want to take the doctors advice about the Digoxin. Part of it was that he told me it would take her about an hour to die, and that it would simulate a heart attack—even though it would not be extraordinarily painful. If I could give her the pain medication and she just went to sleep, maybe it would be better. I knew his concern was primarily for me. He wanted me to be safe, and so he wanted it to be done in whatever way would be the safest thing for me, but I felt really secure. I felt like I don't think you know. My mother was visibly so very badly off that I didn't think anybody was going to say boo (question her dying). And I did not have the same concerns that he had. And I thought I would much rather have my mother go to sleep and die peacefully than to have her go through any more pain.

I just felt very confident there wouldn't be any consequences. Who's going to do an autopsy on an eighty-three-year-old lady, who just came out of the hospital, who has had three strokes this spring and a heart attack? That's ridiculous. Nobody's going to. Oddly enough, even though rationally I recognized that something might go wrong, I think now that I really didn't give enough thought to that possibility, and that's one of the things that I feel that I want to say to other people. Be prepared for something going wrong.

I am extremely fortunate in that I had a friend that I had the confidence to tell about this, and he came to stay with me during this period just to give me moral support. He was coming from out of town, and I was so touched by his coming. This is a very hard thing, and it's hard stress on a friend. It's also a

---

14. Phenophen No. 3 is a mixture of acetaminophen 325 mg plus codeine sulphate 30 mg., both pain-killers. It is stated on p. 1477 of *The Physicians Desk Reference* (35th edition, Medical Economics Company, New Jersey, 1981) the Phenophen No. 3 is "for the relief of mild to moderate pain." Acetaminophen in amounts over 15 grs. is often fatal because of liver damage. Codeine in itself is much more toxic. As stated earlier, the lethal dose of codeine for an adult is approximately "one-half a gram (0.5 gm.) to one gram (1.0 gm.)"—*Clinical Toxicology,* Section II, p. 159. Mary had changed from a not very suitable drug to an even less satisfactory one for self-deliverance.

50

risk for him. I made up my mind to do it before he got here so that he would not have been here when it happened. Just the fact that he was coming made me feel strong enough. So I got up about four or five o'clock in the morning. My mother never appeared to sleep. She'd just be staring. She would take pills if I gave her pills. I could hardly get her to eat, and I was having to give her water with a syringe because I couldn't get her to drink out of a cup. I took one of the pills, and I broke it open and my idea was to dilute them in the water and give them to her with the syringe.

I tasted the powder and it was extremely bitter. Well, my mother could reject what she didn't want. And, I thought, if I put this bitter liquid down her throat as soon as she tastes it, she's going to refuse to take it anymore. She will not swallow. So I think it would be better to give her about fifteen of these capsules. This was sheer guesswork. I had no information; I did not call my doctor friend to ask him. I gave my mother the pills and washed them down with a turkey baster.

I put them in her mouth for she had no coordination at all. She didn't seem to be paralyzed, but she never moved. She'd just stay wherever you put her. Then after I gave her about five of them she turned around and said the first lucid thing she'd said for a week. She looked at me and said, "So many?" My heart just sank and I said, "Yes, Mom." And that was all she needed. She just kept on taking them. When I got to the ninth pill, apparently they had not been going down that well, and one had melted in her mouth and the powder made her throat constrict. I thought, I won't be able to get any more down her, and I was not able to. I had to stop at nine and it was at that point that I got very frightened. Then I sat there and I said to her: "I don't know whether you can understand me or not, it's hard to know what you hear and what you understand, but you told me once that you didn't want to become a vegetable and that you didn't want to go on living in the kind of condition that you're in now. And I made you a promise." I also said, "You're going to sleep now and you won't be in pain anymore." Then I said, "I love you, Mom." And that was the essence of what I said to her. There wasn't any sign at all that she heard me. And then I just sat in a chair in the room and waited.

And what happened was that her respiration became slower and slower. She was taking one breath every twenty seconds and then it became noisy and rasping. I just wanted it to be over. Well, hours later she was still going that same way.

It had been about four or five in the morning when I gave her the pills. Then my friend arrived around noon. And the news I had to greet him with was that I had given my mother the pills but that something had gone wrong and that she had not died. I said, "I'm not exactly sure what to do. I can't call the doctor because they are going to take her to the hospital. I have to see it through and I know I have to finish it. But I'm bewildered now, and I'm frightened, and I don't know exactly what the thing to do is." So he said: "I think you should wait. Your mother doesn't look to me like she's aware of very much." Her eyes looked like pieces of glass, no longer the eyes of a living person.

It was that more than anything that made us think that perhaps at this point she wasn't aware of pain or anything. So we waited and waited and her breath would get slower and then it would get higher, but she was so out of it that I knew that I would not be able to get any liquid into her. I knew I couldn't get pills down her. There wasn't anything I could do. My friend told me to go to bed for awhile, and that he would stay with my mother. Of course, I didn't sleep.

One of the things I started doing—this may seem a little cold-blooded but it actually helped me immeasurably—is that when he went to bed and I got up to watch Mother, I started sitting down at my typewriter and writing out exactly what was going on right then. For instance, my mother right now is doing this and I don't know what to do. Everything, right to the second, of what was happening. When I put it down on that piece of paper it had no fear in it. It had no pain, it was just words on paper and I could see what the facts were. I did that all through the night. And it's amazing, I'll never forget how cold-blooded I felt, and yet I don't know how I would have made the decisions otherwise. It helped me see very clearly what was going on. One of the things that I had to think about was alternatives: I knew I had to finish what I had started. I had to go through these things within myself, through some terrible self-flagellation of a voice within that was saying, "Oh, you were going to do it when it was going to be nice and neat and pretty, and there wasn't going to be anything ugly or unaesthetic, but if you're going to have to do something violent, you know you're not that committed, are you?" I was doing this to myself and saying this because one of the things which had occured to me would be to smother her. This is the decision I ultimately made. I remembered the scene from the movie "One Flew Over the Cuckoo's Nest" when one patient smothers another in the mental hospital because he had been given a lobotomy and was now a vegetable. I remember how violent and ugly that scene was, but also that it was a compassionate scene. It helped me to say to myself, "I can do this also." I held that scene in my head. I said, "This is an act of compassion. It is not an act of brutality."

But one of the decisions I made through the night was that I was not going to do anything so long as I had a feeling of fear. So long as I had the fear in my stomach. Or any of that adrenalin stuff, because I know that fear is a bad way to do anything; it leads you into mistakes, it leads you into poor judgement, and I just thought that whatever I do, as long as I feel fear, I'm not going to do it. And I would go and I would somehow get rid of all the fear. I don't know how I did that. I am a meditator, but I did not meditate that night; this was beyond meditation. But it was like I made a decision: "I'm not going to do anything in fear. This is my mother; this is somebody else's life I'm taking responsibility for. I am not going to do anything when I'm petrified." So I made that decision, and another decision I made was that I was not going to wake up my friend. He had offered me everything a person could offer another person, and now what I offered him was to spare him to have to go through this.

I convinced myself that suffocation is an easy way to go. And I thought, a pillow doesn't seem secure enough to me; if I cut my mother's breath off with something not porous, like a plastic bag, that would be better. I thought this was such a horrid image for me, that I didn't know if I could do that. So I rehearsed. I mean, I was going back and forth to the typewriter and writing all this down, and I got the plastic bag and I went in by my mother's bed. I put it over her face and I held it down and her breath started coming harder. I wasn't ready yet and I pulled it away, but something in me said, "Yes, I can do that. I can do that because I have to."

I went away and sat down again and I wrote some more, and there came a moment where I said, "I'm ready." So I went back with the plastic bag and I held it over my mother's nose and mouth. It wasn't an easy way to go...it's ugly and it's horrible...it took her fifteen minutes to die...and I had to hold that over her face for fifteen minutes and I knew I couldn't let go because I had fouled up once and caused her an additional day of agony. And I could not *not* follow through again. I had to finish. I had to complete it. So I held it down. I just kept on saying, "Forgive me, Mom, forgive me, Mom, forgive me, Mom," over and over again...for fifteen minutes.

I thought her breathing would just go down, and finally she would just sign. Instead her body fought for breath. It was just horrible. My worst agony afterwards was that she had been aware. Now I think not, because she was able to use her hands if she wanted to, but she never did once. Her body thrashed around some, but she never once tried to push my hands away. She did not look at me, her eyes were just staring off, but she was making really horrible, awful sounds. I thought, "I just cannot, cannot withdraw."

There was just no turning back once I had undertaken this act. So I stayed and I kept my finger on the pulse in her neck, and I didn't release the bag until I felt the last beat of her heart.

That's how it went, and that's why I want to contribute this to your book because I don't want anybody else to have to go through that. I don't want the person dying to go through it, and I don't want the person helping to go through it. The thing that I did wrong was not to call my doctor friend back and tell him I wanted to change the plan. It was not until this interview that it really hit me why I didn't call him: it was because I trusted my own judgement more than I trusted his. I was also afraid that our phone calls would be tapped or overheard.

One thing which helped me survive the experience was being able to share it with my friend. He made a special effort to be with me at the time of Mother's death, and since then we have talked about it frequently. Without a sounding board like him, it would have been much harder for me. Talking to you has also helped me clear up a few things in my mind.

I have really put myself through an awful lot of self-examination about the way I approached this and how I could have avoided those mistakes. I finally decided that this society makes it so difficult to even approach this kind of thing that I can't find it in my heart to condemn myself. The society and the system have just made it so insane. One of the problems is that information is not accessible.

What came out of this experience for me was that I had one of those agreements with a friend about this kind of thing, that if either one of us ever became terminally ill, we would help the other. I have now withdrawn from that agreement. I am going to be responsible for my own death; I don't want to put anybody through what I had to go through for my mother. I was willing to do this for her, I am not sorry I went through it, I would do it again, even if things went wrong again, because I think even though things went wrong and she suffered horribly that last day, I probably spared her quite a long time of suffering.

Since she died, I have asked my mother; I have said, "Mother, did I do wrong?" I quite clearly hear her saying, "You did the best you could, you did the best you could. It's all right." I feel forgiveness from her.

She had said to me many times over the course of those months, "I have wanted to die for years." I say, "Now, well then, Mother why didn't you? Why did you put us both through this, why didn't you have the courage? Once again you have been totally dependent, once again you have left all the responsibility to others."

When she had her heart attack, for instance, she called the lady downstairs. She set off at that time a course of events that were inevitable, because the neighbor called the paramedics and of course the medics have to work as hard as they can to save the life. Everybody in the whole system has no choice— they have professional and legal responsibilities; they may also feel that they have a moral responsibility. But the beginning of the responsibility is with the person who called for help. I've made up my mind I'm not asking anybody else to do that for me.

In saying that I am angry with my mother, at the same time I understand that she never had the chance to make a responsible decision. But I think I'm trying more to speak in some kind of metaphor, using my mother as an example. I have forgiven my mother, I understand her situation totally. But I can still be mad at her. Do you know what I mean?

If my mother had only had a chance to think about her death and to talk to me about it long before she had her heart attack, and for her to have some support and say, "Look, if something should happen to me, I don't want to be kept alive." If she had an agreement with a friend, then the friend would just come and stay with her and not call the medics. But, of course, my mother never thought about it at all.

The other place I can see clearly where it got insane is that when she broke her hip they took her out of that nursing home and performed an operation on her hip to put a pin in it. At that point I should have known the doctor well enough. We should have laws which would have allowed him and me to stand and talk and say this: "Your mother has expressed the desire to die, and her case is hopeless; she's going to die in two or three months. Anyway, there's no point in putting her through any more pain. She's broken her hip; let's put her quietly to sleep." It was a nightmare from the beginning, but at that point it was so outrageously insane. Even my mother in her insanity could see it. She just looked at the ambulance drivers and said, "Oh, what's the use?" with so much feeling. "Oh, what's the use? Leave me alone, let me die," she said.

In the last few days, and especially in the last hours before I gave her the medication, a lot of what was going on with me that was so painful was really intense self-examination to see if my motives were pure. And I found out that they were pure. There were all the things I asked myself: Do I just want to get rid of this responsibility? Do I just not want to have to cope with my mother's dying days? And the answers to these questions were, yes, I don't want to put myself through this, and I want to relieve my own suffering. I said, Are you doing this to relieve your own suffering? Yes, I am. It's something that I'm going through in all areas of my life, through my middle age, and that is realizing that my motivations for doing things are never all one thing or another. They're never all good and all bad; they're never all pure nor all malicious. They are always mixed.

Although I could find elements of all these things in my feelings, the overriding one was of compassion for my mother. And I knew with such a rockhard certainty that I loved my mother as I had never loved her in all my life that I had to trust that. I could not for mean motives kill my mother when I felt such love for her. It wouldn't be possible to have those two things. If we are honest with ourselves, we can find little selfish and mean motives for everything. So it was really good to admit that they were in there because then I didn't feel like I was untrue to myself or fooling myself. It was really actually a relief when I wrote down in that journal, "Are you doing this so that you don't have to go through the agony?" And to say, "Yes." I could look at that and say, "Oh, good, I can say that." The central thing was this love that I felt and the memory of mother's intensely expressed desire to die, something she repeated several times over those months.

Ever since then I have looked at people who before I might have feared, and I have this little statement I can make in my head. "If I can kill my own mother, I can do anything and you don't scare me." It sounds really cockamamie, but it is true. It took so much courage that now I feel I cannot justify being cowardly ever again in my life. If I could do that then I have no excuse for not confronting anything and everything that frightens me. That's a great strength that has come to me through this.

CHAPTER SEVEN

The sense of death is most in apprehension.

Whether rational suicide should be available to everyone is not an argument which this book is addressing. Some philosophers have argued that suicide is a basic human right; others have declared that it is incompatible with the Christian ethic and/or that it is an act of supreme selfishness.

Whatever one's view, the fact remains that suicide is endemic in our society and always has been. (Professor Larue, in his appendix to this book, deals with the historical and cultural aspects of suicide.) Hemlock is concerned, as are many reasonable people, that more be done to prevent unnecessary suicides of people intent on destroying themselves because of temporary unhappiness or an unbalanced state of mind. It is particularly distressing to see the increasing number of youth suicides both in Europe and North America and we, for example, encourage programs which guide parents and others in detecting any of the symptoms signalling impending suicide in young people.

As stated earlier, Hemlock is arguing for the rights of the advanced terminally ill and the seriously incurably ill to have the option of rational suicide (or, to use the term we prefer, self-deliverance). These are people who are going to die soon and of known causes anyway.

The argument we make for self-deliverance, however, is clouded by the notoriety of the act of suicide in the public mind. In the past forty years the news media has felt free to be much more explicit in reporting the seamier side of life, and one of the results of this openness is that suicides of a particularly gruesome nature have been reported (or are those remembered). Thus suicide often has a connotation of a sinister, degrading act when even its strongest opponents would have to agree that, however rare, it is not always so.

Of course, putting obstructions in the way of potential suicides is one way to prevent compulsive, unnecessary self-destruction. Where there is enough determination, however, no obstacle can deter a truly suicidal person. The following instances testify to a remarkable ingenuity. For example, there has been: drowning from placing one's head in a toilet bowl, drowning from placing one's head in a bathroom or kitchen sink, falling or jumping from a flagpole or telephone pole, falling or jumping from statues, bridges, monuments, or trees, jumping from a moving train, jumping from an airplane without a parachute, jumping into an elevator shaft, discharging gunshot wounds to different parts of the body, inflicting fatal burns on oneself by setting oneself afire (immolation), placing one's head in the oven and turning on the gas, fatal burns from placing oneself in hot water in a bathtub or shower, overexposure to cold weather, suffocation from placing oneself in an empty refrigerator, suffocation from enclosure in an airtight room or closet, starvation, electrocution from touching the inside of electrical appliances while switched on, electrocution from touching exposed wires and elecrical wires and electrical objects with wet hands, poisoning oneself from swallowing disinfectants, cleansing fluids, or other household products such as insecticides, or fatal self-stabbing by a sharp and cutting instrument such as a knife, broken glass, or razor.

There are, in addition to the above, other ways in which people have ended their lives while simultaneously trying to simulate an accident. These have included: overexposure or an extended stay in a sauna bath or steam bath, falling from a trampoline while jumping on it, falling in front of a train or other moving vehicle, fatal burns from a fire deliberately started inside a parked automobile, fatal burns suffered from hot compresses, asphyxiation from an earth cave-in or self-burial, driving a car into a pole or wall or over a cliff, an intentional nosedive by a pilot of an aircraft, an industrial "accident" in which an individual jumps from a higher level to a lower one in the course of performing a job, an industrial "accident" in which an individual is crushed by equipment or machinery he is operating, an attack resulting from intentional contact with wild or untrained animals, or a fatal blow resulting from a heavy falling object which one purposefully places himself in the path of.

One method of suicide frequently used, and thus much publicized, has been the use of fumes from a car exhaust. Those who have carried it out successfully have first made sure that they have had complete privacy for several hours; they have had the car checked for smooth and reliable engine running, with the idle slightly accelerated. They have also ensured that the fuel tank was full. Using a hose, often taken from a domestic vacuum cleaner, they extended the tube through a window in the car, with the gaps at the side blocked by stuffing them with rags, allowing some ventilation by lowering another window about an inch so that the gases could circulate. The carbon monoxide in the car's exhaust fumes was lethal if inhaled in large enough quantities; the lethality came from the combination of the carbon monoxide with oxygen-carrying hemoglobin in the blood, depriving the brain or oxygen.

People using this method have usually reckoned that the smell was repulsive, and many have feared choking. To avoid such unpleasantness, they took a large quantity of alcohol and/or drugs (invariably barbituates) before switching on the ignition.

On the "60 Minutes" CBS television program in October, 1980, a demonstration was given of how a man who had been a double agent for the U.S. Government appeared to have committed suicide by self-electrocution in a motel room. He had, it was shown, run a bare wire around his chest and connected the ends to an electrical outlet; he then sat on a chair with his thumb in a cup of water and switched on the power.[15]

---

15. "When the heart is a component of the electrical pathway (circuit) the effect may be lethal...Domestic house current (A.C.) of 100 volts with low cycles (about 60 Hz) is dangerous to the heart, since it may cause ventricular fibrillation." *Current Medical Diagnosis and Treatment,* p. 945.

Others have chosen to die by lying in a bath of water and then dropping a live wire into the water. Some of these people have elected to take an overdose of drugs and a substantial amount of alcohol as well, although occasionally this led to failures since unconsciousness set in before the wire was dropped into the water. More thoughtful people have left a sign indicating that the electric current should be switched off before they were touched.

Some individuals have drowned themselves in their own baths, taking a heavy dose of drugs to ensure unconsciousness, and then turning on the tap so that it ran slowly until the bath was filled with water. In many cases this method failed because the overflow outlet was too low to permit the body to be fully immersed, or the continuous running of water from the overflow alerted neighbors.

Among the infinite variety of ways in which people have tried to end their lives, a common method has been the cold bath. In this instance hypothermia was caused when the body temperature dropped several degrees below the normal figure of thiry-seven (37) centigrade. Initally there is a loss of consciousness, and as the body temperature continues to drop over the next few hours, death follows. Usually the person attempting this stepped into a slightly warmed bath and left the cold tap running. Again, consumption of a large amount of drink and drugs has often taken place to make the act more bearable since it requires at least an hour to be effective. In cold climates, people using this method of self-destruction have accelerated death by opening a window and permitting cold air to accumulate.[16]

In countries near the Arctic Circle, hypothermia is a fairly common form of suicide. Two methods are used. One way is to take sleeping pills or antidepressants and lie down in the snow to sleep never to awake. Another way is to jump into the sea in order to die from a combination of cold and drowning.

Another common method—not always successful—has been overdosing on aspirin. Swallowed in massive quantities, the overdose has proven lethal in some instances, but it has taken hours to upset the body's chemistry and has had many unpleasant side-effects, such as heavy bleeding of the stomach, nausea and dizziness. For people who have attempted suicide in this way, because aspirin is not a sedative, it did not induce unconsciousness while its chemicals were taking effect. The method used was not a particularly painless one. Similarly, Paracetamol (not a sedative either) when taken in huge doses, has caused serious inflammation of the liver which has sometimes—but not always—proved fatal. Paracetamol is another name for acetaminophen.

Slashing throats and wrists has only worked in the past if people have had extremely sharp weapons and some knowledge of anatomy guaranteeing the severance of vital arteries. Many people who have sought self-destruction in

---

16. "Immersion in cold water can also cause a rapid fall in the victim's core temperature, so that systemic hypothermia and death may occur before actual drowning." *Current Medical Diagnosis and Treatment,* p. 944.

this way have ended up cutting tendons and nerves and were left alive but disabl-ed. Bleeding to death has also been most distressing both to the individuals and to those who have discovered them. People who have hanged themselves have often done so as an act of revenge against someone else, for the shock of fin-ding a garrotted person is one of the worst experiences that could be inflicted by one human being upon another.

The methods of self-destruction mentioned above have all been effective in some instances—with some judgement and some luck—but they have also been known to fail. With careful planning and forethought, people using them have succeeded in dying, but the main disadvantage in such techniques is that they are not likely to appeal to the advanced terminally ill person, either practically or aesthetically.

On balance, the methods of suicide described here are too gruesome for people who embrace Hemlock's philosophy. Therefore we will describe how people have carried out more distinguished forms of self-deliverance.

Footnote: The 'natural gas' used in today's cooking ovens is *not* lethal, as was the old 'city gas'.

CHAPTER EIGHT

All substances are poisons; there is none which is not a poison.
The right dose differentiates a poison and a remedy.

—PARACELUS (1493-1541)

Many terminally ill people have wanted to practice self-deliverance properly, like the parents of Mary McFee and Frank Robinson, but have found themselves unable to do so because of ignorance or non-availability of a suitable method. Even a few physicians and scientists, who should have known better despite their illness, have procrastinated and found themselves seriously incapacitated before securing the necessary means to accelerate their death.

The Hemlock Society welcomes the day when an attending physician can, without fear of penalty, be asked to supply the means of self-deliverance for a rational terminally ill person. Of course, a physician should have the right to refuse to help in hastening death if his conscience forbids it, but he should be obliged to refer the request to a colleague who is willing. Until this time comes, however, most individuals who want voluntary euthanasia must fend for themselves.

In the past the most successful practice of voluntary euthanasia has been with the use of drugs. While secret service agencies like the C.I.A. and the K.G.B. have their James Bond-like, three-second pills with which to wipe out themselves or one other, such sophisticated tools of self-destruction are not available to the public.

After his arrest in 1945, Heinrich Himmler, the head of the S.S. in Nazi Germany, killed himself with a vial of potassium cyanide which he had concealed in a cavity in his gums. He died within twelve minutes of biting on it although efforts were made to pump his stomach and administer emetics. Hermann Goering also avoided the hangman by taking a similar poison which was smuggled into his cell. Few poisons are faster-acting that cyanide or, to use its other name, prussic acid. Only between sixty and ninety miligrams (60 to 90 mg.) are required to kill a human.[17] Whilst cyanide is a most effective poison—perhaps the most effective—the intense pain of the dying should not be underestimated. The pain may be brief—depending on the quantity ingested—but it is appaling. For this reason believers in voluntary euthanasia would not recommend it because the essence of the concept is a painless and non-violent death which loved ones ought, if they wish, to be present at. In those states of the U.S.A. which have carried out executions in gas chambers, the pellets used were hydrogen cyanide, which kills in a very short time when inhaled.

Yet it has been found that some of the drugs stored in domestic medicine cabinets from previous illnesses or periods of stress were perfectly effective if used in the correct lethal doses and accompanied by the right intake of food and liquid. As was the case with Sonia Hertz and Jean Humphry, a light meal

---

17. *Clinical Toxicology of Commercial Products,* Section III, p. 106.

was most productive in facilitating drug ingestion; both women were aware that an empty stomach could hasten absorption of drugs into the system, but that it also intensified the risk of vomiting. On the other hand, a heavy meal could delay absorption considerably. They deliberately ate a light snack (tea and toast) an hour before pill-taking, the most conducive interval.

Experiments have shown that another way to reduce the risk of vomiting has been to take a travel sickness pill one hour before the drug-taking, usually with the light meal. (The most careful practitioners of self-deliverance have first tested, over the previous days, whether the pill has induced drowsiness which might, of course, prevent them from taking the main dose later on.) It has also been found by people taking large doses of drugs that the simultaneous drinking of soda water hastens absorption of the pills into one's system.

(See special footnote at end of chapter on antiemetics.)

Certainly the public has been warned innumerable times that drinking alcohol while taking sleeping pills is dangerous. A combination with narcotics or barbiturates may be lethal, and ignorance of this fact has cost many lives. According to the writers of *The Prediction of Suicide:* "When any ingestion is accompanied by alcohol, increase the strength-count (of the drugs) by fifty per cent."

The combined fatal dose can sometimes be even less that that. Wallace B. Mendelson says in his book on sleeping pills: "Studies on the interaction of barbiturates and ethanol (alcohol) show a relatively consistent, often fatal, enhancement of toxic effects. When taken together, blood concentrations as low as one-half a milligram (0.5 mg.) per 100 milliliters (ml.) of secobarbital and 100 milligrams (mg.) per 100 milliliters (ml.) of ethanol may prove fatal; in contrast, fatal levels of secobarbital taken alone range from one and one tenth (1.1) to six (6.0) mg. per 100 milliliters (ml.) and those of ethanol are thought to be in the range of at least 400 milligrams (mg.) per 100 milliliters.[18](Secobarbital is the generic name for Seconal).

The maximum effect of the interaction of drugs and drinks can be achieved by taking undiluted spirits as slowly as possible after ingesting the lethal dose of drugs.

Physicians are, of course, acutely aware of this combination. As the editor of the medical magazine *Lancet* commented in an editorial in the September 13, 1980, issue: "In medical profession, the suicide rate is high, and one wonders how much this has to do with access to painless lethal agents. A favorite medical method is said to be whiskey and a bottle of barbiturates in a parked car."

Physicians also know that barbiturates will not leave them mentally impaired should their suicide attempt fail. "Usually recovery from barbiturate coma is

---

18. *The Use and Misuse of Sleeping Pills* by Wallace B. Mendelson, M.D. (Plenum Medical Book Company, New York & London, 1980), p. 116.

without neurologic deficit even after severe poisoning.... The rarity of permanent damage after barbiturate coma contrasts with the not infrequent sequelae to carbon monoxide poisoning," say Casarett and Doull.[19]

Some people concerned with careful planning preferred to remove the powdered drug from the capsule and pour it into a liquid. As was the case with Sonia Hertz and Jean Humphry, it was found that this could (and should) be done with as little liquid as possible and as close to the intended time of ingestion as was convenient. To improve the bitter taste of the pills, people have added coffee, honey, or other flavored substances at the last minute. The Harley Street physician who prescribed the lethal dose for Jean Humphry wanted death to occur as quickly as possible and thus recommended combined overdoses of Seconal (secobarbital) and Codeine (a derivative of opium), which together caused acute depression of the central nervous system and precipitated death within fifty minutes. Typically, the fastest and most potent combinations of drugs to which lay people have reasonable access have been barbituates (sleeping pills) taken with analgesics (pain killers). "Overdose with hypnotic [sedative] drugs," states the Merck Manual of Diagnosis and Therapy, "remains the most common form of suicide by drug ingestions."[20]

According to Goodman and Gilman, "The lethal dose of a barbituate varies with many factors and cannot be stated with certainty. Severe poisoning is likely to occur when more than ten times the full hypnotic dose has been ingested at once. The barbituates with short half-lives and high lipid solubility are more potent and more toxic than the more polar, long-acting compounds such as phenobarbital and barbital. The potentially fatal dose of phenobarbital is six to ten grams (6 to 10 gm.), whereas that of amobarbital and secobarbital or pentobarbital is two to three grams (2 to 3 gm.)"[21]

A differing view of the dosage with respect to phenobarbital is presented in the book, *Justifiable Euthanasia*,[22] which gives information to physicians in the Netherlands about helping terminally ill patients to die. Dr. Admiraal, the author, states that the lethal dose of phenobarbital is between four and six grams (4 to 6 gm.), and he puts the lethal dose of amobarbital, pentobarbital and secobarbital at between six and eight grams (6 to 8 gm.) when taken orally.

In the toxicity chart of the thirty drugs most frequently used in suicide attempts given in *The Prediction of Suicide* the *minimum* lethal dose of butabarbital and pentobarbital is stated as one gram (1 gm.), and that of secobarbital,

---

19. *Toxicology: The Basic Science of Poisons,* 2nd edition, by Casarett and Doull, (Macmillan, New York, 1980), p. 191.

20. (Merck and Co., Rahway, New Jersey, 13th edition), p. 1853.

21. *The Pharmacological Basis of Therapeutics,* p. 359.

22. *Justifiable Euthanasia: A Guide for Physicians,* by Dr. P.V. Admiraal, (The Netherlands Voluntary Euthanasia Society, Amsterdam, 1981), p. 11.

amobarbital and phenobarbital as one and one half grams (1.5 gm.).

(Note: Seconal is secobarbital, Amytal is amobarbital, Carbrital and Nembutal are pentobarbital, Tuinal is amo-secobarbital, Butisol (Soneryl in Europe) is butabarbital, Luminal is phenobarbital.)

Students of these two books have been careful to note that Dr. Admiraal is giving the lethal dosage to cover all types of cases and body weights, while the second book is indicating the *smallest* dosage which *can* kill, especially if alcohol is taken. The weight and bulk of each person is an important factor in deciding appropriate doses. In addition, one must consider whether someone has been taking the same, or similar, drugs for some time and has thus built up a tolerance to the substance. A small, frail person such as Sonia Hertz needed only the minimum lethal dose to kill her.

In its list of minimum lethal dosages, *The Prediction of Suicide* states that as little as one half a gram (.5 gm.) of Percodan can be fatal, while the same goes for one and two-tenths (1.2 gm.) of Demerol and two grams (2 gm.) of Darvon*. Copies of this book's toxicity chart have been circulated all over the world by people in the voluntary euthanasia movements, but they have always been careful to advise that the given minimum lethal dose should be multiplied by at least three to ensure lethality.

It is useful to know that 1,000 milligrams (mg.) equals fifteen grains (15 gr.) which equals one gram (gm.). For example, to ingest six grams requires the consumption of sixty tablets each of one hundred milligrams (mg.) Another way of expressing this dosage is: 60 by 100 mg. or merely 60 x 100.

Generally, the use of analgesics (painkillers) alone has not been recommended for self-deliverance, although some people in desperation have effectively used two grams (2 gm.) of Codeine together with alcohol and a few tranquilizers such as Valium** or Librium.

Another last resort for some people practicing voluntary euthanasia has been the consumption of the non-barbiturate, non-benzodiazepine hypnotics, the best known of which is methaqualone marketed under the brand name of Quaalude in the U.S.A. and Mandrax in Europe. These drugs relieve anxiety and tension and also induce sleep. It is known that, whereas an overdose of barbiturates and narcotic drugs induces sleep, and subsequently death, through depression of the central nervous system, these particular hypnotics act something like aspirin, and they promote severe and unpleasant damage to the stomach, liver and kidneys. According to *The Use and Misuse of Sleeping Pills,* (p. 94), the estimated fatal dose of Doriden, Quaalude, and Nodular is five grams (5 gm.), but is as low as two grams (2 gm.) for Chloral hydrate triclofos (Triclos).

There has been a great deal of publicity recently about certain non-prescription,

---

* Darvon has gained a reputation for quick lethality in self-deliverance. Two grams (30 tablets of 65 mg each) are required. Beware that Darvon (generic name propoxyphene) is NOT a sleep agent so one should be included for peaceful self-deliverance.

**Valium by itself will not effect self-deliverance of a dying person. An overdose of 500 mg (100 tablets of 5 mg each) is lethal provided it is combined with plenty of strong alcohol and/or narcotic or barbiturate drugs.)

or "over-the-counter" drugs which are rumored to be lethal if taken in suffi cient quantities. So far as Hemlock's research can tell, the only one reported to be effective (theoretically, at any rate) was the travel-sickness drug, Pro methazine, commercially known as Phenergan (or Avomine in Europe). No case has come to public attention as an example of self-deliverance using this drug, possibly because the lethal dose has been listed by one physician[23] as six grams, which he pointed out meant consuming 240 of the twenty-five milligram tablets (240 x 25 mg.). This is probably impossible—or certainly difficult—to achieve before losing consciousness.

It has also become widely known that anti-depressant tablets taken in massive quantity can be lethal. These drugs have been described as "tricyclic" and af fect the nervous system producing a limited psychic effect. Considering the cases reported to us, the minimum lethal dose averaged out to be five grams.

It is interesting to note that in the Dutch manual for doctors on euthanasia *(Justifiable Suicide)*, all drugs to be used—except for the barbituates—were to be given by intravenous, intra-muscular, or sub-cutaneous injection. Barbituates were the only drug recommended to be taken orally.

A private study of the suicides of anaesthetists in Florida indicated that almost all of the physicians who killed themselves did so by using an intravenous injec tion of one gram of Pentothal (which in Europe has the generic name of Thiopen tal and is often marketed under the name of Nesdonal). Pentothal is widely us ed by veterinarians to put sick or injured animals to sleep. This is a strictly con trolled drug and available only to the medical profession.

Those few people with access to arsenic—usually pharmacists or physicians— have found that the fatal dose was somewhere between one-tenth (0.1) and one- half (0.5) a gram, but because death could take up to forty-eight hours, it has not been a favored drug for voluntary euthanasia. It is extremely difficult to obtain as well since arsenic toxide is nearly tasteless and odorless, and has been frequently used in the past by persons whose motives in putting someone else to death have been anything but compassionate. Consequently it is almost im possible to obtain on the open market.

We are often asked about the use of hemlock, and for obvious reasons! We use the name to represent our society because of its symbolism and its well-known connection with Socrates. Historians report that in ancient Greece magistrates kept some hemlock in court and offered it to anyone who was suffering from a terminal illness, or who had asked the judiciary to be permitted to commit suicide rather than suffer punishment and disgrace. It is not recommended by pharmacologists today, however; it causes painful reaction and dying takes place over several hours. The ingredient in hemlock which actually kills is Coniine, and while consumption of 100 milligrams has been known to be fatal, others

---

23. Dr. George Mair in *How to Die With Dignity*, p. 29. Other textbooks do not mention a minimum lethal dose, while the *Clinical Toxicology of Commercial Products* rates pro methazine as "slightly toxic" (p. 222).

have tolerated up to 150 milligrams without undue discomfort.

People such as Mary McFee's mother who have been prescribed Digoxin for heart complaints have made attempts to end their lives with the drug. Dosages of more than ten milligrams (10 mg.) have generally been lethal (the actual lethal range of the drug has been listed as between ten and twenty milligrams).[24] Strychnine, another famous poison, has been known to induce death within an hour, but only after violent convulsions. The fatal dose taken orally is anywhere from 100 to 120 milligrams,[25] but the effects are so unpleasant that most people prefer something more gentle and soporific.

How have so many people intent on taking their own lives been able to secure the drugs mentioned above, and in large enough quantities to ensure a swift, certain death?

The answer is: it has not always been easy. The first place many have looked is, rightly enough, one's own medicine cabinet. (California's Narcotic Authority estimates that the average family has about two bottles of legally prescribed drugs left over from an illness.)[26] If there were sufficient barbiturates and analgesics there, the first question was whether their strength (toxicity) had deteriorated with time. The answer many of them found—or guessed at—was probably the drugs had not been spoiled.

Manufacturers tend to "play safe" by stating on their labels only half the true life of a drug. In fact, nearly all drugs last up to three years, and barbiturates up to eight years. Some people, aware of this fact, have carefully stored drugs for years in preparation for the day when they would want to use them should they contract a terminal illness. Gelatine capsules tend to decompose after a year, so some individuals protected their effectivenesss by emptying the powder from the capsules into a small, dry, brown bottle, tightly sealing it, and placing it in a darkened, cool place where no child or house guest could get access.

The gelatine capsules, by the way, react quite strongly to alcohol, which is another reason why a combination of drugs and drink is often fatal. The principle on which many drugs are meant to work is that the gelatine decomposes in the body slowly, and the drug is released into the body little by little. As a famous magazine has pointed out: "The tiny time pills found in capsules are slow to release their active ingredients and are meant to be absorbed gradually. The outer covering of these pills is often quite soluble in alcohol. The result may be that instead of receiving the drug over eight or twelve hours, you may

---

24. *The Clinical Toxicology of Commercial Products,* Section II, pp. 164-65.

25. *The Clinical Toxicology of Commercial Products,* Section III, p. 303.

26. "Your family's medicine chest may be the source of illicit drugs." Los Angeles Times, March 15, 1981.

get a whopping dose all at once and experience toxic effects."[27]

Some people have built up a supply of medication by saving a few strong drugs from every prescription given over the years. Others have gone to their doctors, asked for sleeping pills and then have not used them. Europeans often acquire drugs during holidays in Spain and Italy, where barbituates are more liberally prescribed by doctors, especially to a tourist with foreign currency who complains of not sleeping because of heat, noise or strange surroundings. Many doctors in Mexico will also prescribe barbiturates in these circumstances, requiring payment in dollars.

Pharmacists tell me it is the older doctors who today mostly prescribe barbiturates (Seconal, Tuninal, etc.) as sleeping aids. Younger doctors barely know these drugs and invariably prescribe *the more harmless* benzodiazepines such as Dalmane as relaxants.

Hemlock has learned of people of the utmost respectability buying drugs from street pushers in New York and Los Angeles (to name just two cities) in order to help a dying friend who wanted release from his or her suffering. Needless to say such action required considerable courage and devotion. To wander alone into what may be a high-crime area and use the appropriate street jargon is not an easy task.[28] First they had to learn what to ask for, using appropriate street jargon such as "Big Reds" (Seconal) and "Rainbows" (Tuinal). Experience has shown, however, that it is unwise to buy heroin or cocaine through a random "pusher" because of its uncertain quality.

Cautious planners have also observed that many serious ill patients are already having their pain controlled by derivatives of cocaine[29] and heroin and have thus built up a tolerance.

The main criticism of the first two editions of this book was that it did not inform the believer in voluntary euthanasia about where the lethal drugs, which would gently ease into death a terminally-ill suffer, could be obtained. There is still no simple answer—perhaps it is a safeguard against untimely, ill-considered suicides that there is not?—but the following are the guide-lines which the Hemlock Society from experience can offer on securing the means:—

---

27. "Danger! These drug combinations may kill you." *Good Housekeeping,* April, 1981, p. 236.

28. James Long lists the street names of drugs in *The Essential Guide to Prescription Drugs.*

29. "In a nonaddicted adult who is not in pain, sixty milligrams (60 mg.) of morphine is generally a toxic dose; one hundred milligrams (100 mg.) is always dangerous, and the probable lethal dose lies between 120 mg. and 250 mg. (2 to 4 grains)," says *The Clinical Toxicology of Commercial Products,* Section III, p. 238. "The minimum lethal dose of cocaine is sometimes said to be one point two grams (1.2 gm.), but death has resulted from application of thirty milligrams (30 mg.) to the nasal mucous membranes." *Current Medical Diagnosis and Treatment,* p. 970.

. Do not consider using non-prescriptions drugs. They are painful and unreliable. The Hemlock Society cannot supply drugs. 2. Check your medicine cabinet for unused barbiturates. 3. Tell your own physician about your belief in voluntary euthanasia to test his reactions. It often helps to say (if it is so) that you are a member of the Hemlock Society. 4. Either at that point, or a little later, calmly ask your physician if he would help you to die when your life is ebbing away and if you wished to accelerate the end. Beware of bland assurances such as 'I'll see you don't suffer at the end.'' 5. Come to an understanding with your physician about exactly what he would or would not do. Ask him outright for a prescription for 40 Seconal, hinting that if he gave you 20 capsules this month and 20 next he would not be accused of prescribing a fatal overdose. Judging from intelligence passed to us from members, this approach sometimes works. Remember, suicide is not a crime and even if the doctor is obstructive there is nothing he can do about it. And it is preferable that he knows your thoughts even if he remains unco-operative. 6. Try asking other doctors the same question. You may be agreeably surprised at the response from one of them. 7. If all else has failed tell a doctor that you cannot sleep and that mild sedatives such as Dalmane definitely do not help. Be firm. If necessary, accept small amounts of barbiturates and start a hoard. 8. When on holiday, especially abroad, try the "can't sleep" ploy. A doctor is less likely to worry about consequences when prescribing for a foreigner. 9. When talking to friends of the same philosophical persuasion, ask them if they have found a doctor who is co-operative. They do exist. 10. Remember that a doctor has his (or her) legal and ethical problems to consider. These are riskier for some than for others. First responses to your pleas may be cool. Tactfully try again later. With some doctors, the timing of the hand-over of the overdose is crucial. Weigh that consideration. Be patient.

The health professions use the word emetic when they mean vomiting. For assured anti-emetic control, an antihistamine and a phenothiazine may be desirable. Onset of the action is from 30 to 60 minutes, with peak effect in one or two hours. They may be taken with food or milk, but not with antacids which will interfere with their absorption. Here are the names of the most effective and most widely used:

PHENOTHIAZINES

Generic name	Brand name
PROCHLORPERAZINE	compazine
CHLORPROMAZINE	thorazine
TRIFLUOPERAZINE	stelazine
PERPHENAZINE	trilafon

Antihistamines

DIMENHYDRINATE	dramamine
MECLIZINE	bonine
CYCLIZINE	marezine
DIPHENHYDRAMINE	benadryl

Two phenothiazines are available in suppository form: Prochlorperazine (compazine) and Promethzine (phenergan). The one major phenothizine which also has some significant antihistaminic properties is promethazine (Phenergan). If you have had travel sickness pills in your medicine cabinet for some years, first check on their lifespan.

CHAPTER NINE

Dying,
Is an art like everything else.
I do it exceptionally well.

—SYLVIA PLATH

The choice of whether an act of self-deliverance is to be conducted alone or in the presence of a loved one or friend has always been an intensely personal one. Many people have already made up their minds on this matter, but for those who have not, it may be helpful to discuss the options that have faced others.

Rational suicide for the advanced terminally ill and the seriously incurably ill requires, above all, seclusion. A grieviously sick person often has little solitude, which is no bad thing, of course, as people comfort the anguish and help administer pain controls. But there is scant chance that a person in this state can secure total, unrelieved privacy.

Certainly it has been found to be nearly impossible to terminate one's own life in a hospital. The task of the medical staff being to care for and treat the dying person (often to the exclusion of everything else), watchfulness is their duty. More than one physician has commented to Hemlock that, whereas voluntary euthanasia could be carried out in the past as a kind of pact between doctor and patient, because of the abundance of safeguards and technical monitoring systems in many hospitals today, it is no longer possible. The instant a life is threatened—or ceases—buzzers go off to alert the resuscitation teams.

In addition, given the present state of the laws on assisted suicide, it is perhaps unfair to involve a physician or nurse in even the most rational and justified suicide. In 1980 there were at least three cases in which nurses in the U.S.A. were charged with the murder or manslaughter of grieviously sick patients, whilst in 1983 two physicians in Los Angeles have faced murder charges.

Thus people considering self-deliverance have to make an extremely difficult decision either not to go into a hospital or to discharge themselves from one so that they can have control over their own destinies, even if it deprives them of some of the advantages of hospital treatment.

It takes courage and determination to cut short one's existence as the one sure way to take command of the medical situation; it takes even more sensitivity to make individual assessments about the quality of one's life. Timing is the most difficult aspect of intelligent voluntary euthanasia, and practical considerations are important: Am I really terminally ill? Should I get a second opinion on my medical prognosis? (A wise person will have considered these last two questions earlier in the treatment.) The two crucial qualitative questions are: How much longer will I live? When is enough?

Christiaan Barnard defines the criteria for deciding as being much more than one's vital signs or physiology. One's value system is crucial, "the whole conglomeration of sensual experiences that the patient calls 'being alive'—the experiences that by their very complexity and subtlety are not amenable to measurement or statistical analysis and are usually known only to the patient, his closest associates and his doctor."[30] And, of course, a key question is also: Will I be considered irrational if I do not make my move until I am critically ill and considered past reason and good judgement?

There has been widespread comment and some criticism of the New York artist, Jo Roman, that at the point in 1979 when she took her life with four and a half (4.5 gm.) grams of Seconal, she was not what doctors would classify as terminally ill. On the basis of the television program about her dying, I at first felt inclined to agree with the criticism, but after reading her book, *Exit House*, [31] I could better understand her logic. Her malignant cancer was well advanced when first discovered, and chemotherapy made her extremely ill and uncomfortable. Mrs. Roman reasoned that two-thirds of the quality of her life was being destroyed by the chemotherapy, so she stopped the treatment. She then set a date for her self-deliverance, something which was undeniably her lawful right and a fundamental moral and civil liberty. Mrs. Roman ended her life with considerable dignity—and with the consent of her family, whom she did not involve in the final act.

A lesson we can learn from Mrs. Roman's experience is the importance of careful consideration and planning well in advance. Perhaps, therefore, the most significant underlying reason for joining a voluntary euthanasia society while still healthy is to signal to one's family and associates that this philosophy has been considered and accepted and should therefore be respected in an emergency.

It's an obvious point—but one often overlooked for whatever reasons—that people who have decided to die alone because illness has made their life unbearable must decide to act before becoming absolutely dependent on others. It is necessary to decide in advance on the method and secure the means, and then act when there is no risk of interference. The means must therefore be fairly fast-acting and, as our stories have indicated, with drugs this is not always so. (Of course, if a person has decided to use a gun, these difficulties do not arise. But I have probably talked to more people intending voluntary euthanasia than most and have yet to meet one who plans their eventual death by shooting. A very few have decided on the car exhaust method.)

People electing to use a solitary method of self-deliverance must also consider the stunning effect their death has on loved ones who suddenly discover

30. *Good Life, Good Death: A Doctor's Case for Euthanasia and Suicide,* (Prentice-Hall Inc., New Jersey, 1980), p. viii.

31. *Exit House: Choosing Suicide as an Alternative,* by Jo Roman. (Seaview Books, New York, 1980).

them. There is the added trauma of interruption, when someone stumbles un-wittingly on an intended act of self-deliverance and the person is not yet dead. For example, one woman told me: "My husband, suffering from terminal cancer, attempted to end his life by cutting his wrists. I, in a sudden shock, called an ambulance and saved his life. This is my greatest regret. He stayed bodily alive only to suffer months of agony as a sedated vegetable."

Considerate people choosing, or having no other alternative than to die alone, leave a letter apologizing for the shock of their unexpected death and explain-ing their motives. Some suicides in hotels, for instance, have thoughtfully left notes to the staff expressing regret for the trauma and inconvenience caused.

The reasons for wishing to die alone sometimes lie in the soul of the individual, but this solitary act often has a practical and caring basis in not wanting loved ones to feel guilt and possible remorse afterwards for having, however remote-ly, shared in the act. Not involving them also keeps them clear of the criminal law. Such lofty ideals can only command our respect.

Then there is the group of people who have no one to help them to die. At meetings which I address, I am frequently asked by elderly men and women: "Jean had you to help her. I am totally alone. What do I do?" Of all the ques-tions which are put to me in public, this is the one I find most difficult to answer. The most helpful response can only be, I feel, that a person contemplating justified self-deliverance who has no immediate support network must have the temerity to ask among their circle of friends and acquaintances. They may be surprised to find that there is one who has the love, compassion and strength of character to provide some form of support. "Cometh the hour, cometh the man," goes the old saying.

People who have suffered great trials and tribulations frequently tell me that they were astonished at how many good friends they discovered they had once they had communicated their needs. "My friends came out of the woodwork," one of the women mentioned in a previous chapter told me. Another said, "As death approaches for me, I never knew I had so many friends."

It is a common failing to underestimate the quality of one's friendships, for they are so seldom tested.

When my first wife died, she asked me to share with her the moment when she took the lethal dose. I have never had any regrets. I am often asked if I feel any guilt at the part I played, and I truthfully answer that I do not. It was a rich and memorable experience to share her final hours as she prepared for death. Since that occasion in 1975, I have discussed this aspect of dying with hundreds of people in different countries and come to the conclusion that most people do indeed want someone at their side as they go to their death. Some feel very positively that this will be the most meaningful and important moment of companionship in their lives.

For those who have a willing friend or loved one, the request made is that they will be on hand at some crucial time. Sometimes the person has sat in the room while the drugs were taken (as I did); others have chosen to sit in the next room and guard the door against unexpected or unwanted intruders, or merely be present in the house or apartment should something go wrong. Whatever the arrangement and relationship between the two people, often the "angel of mercy" has been provided with a handwritten letter absolving them from complicity or blame under the law, not at all a bad idea.

Certainly there can be nothing more horrendous than a deserved and well-thought-out self-deliverance being thwarted by a caller. For instance, one man told me: "My brother, a doctor, gave my mother sleeping pills, which she took with my agreement to end her life. But they were not strong enough, and a local G.P. came in unexpectedly and revived her. Instead of being sympathetic, he gave her a very bad time, not understanding how ill she was. She died three months later after a terrible time." This is not to imply that all doctors would act thus, but in this age when it is so hard to have a personal physician, how does one know how medical people will react? Then there is the general fear that most doctors have of legal entanglements.

From all the experiences told me by other people who have been involved in self-deliverance, it cannot be stressed enough that there must be an *explicit* understanding between the people involved as to what is intended. Such phrases as, "You will help me, won't you?" and "When the time comes I can depend on you, can't I?" have frequently been known to be misunderstood at the eleventh hour. Vague assurances of assistance are easily reneged on, especially when extreme pressure, emotional upheaval and the fear of guilt are involved. Make any agreements extremely clear and specific.

Couples or close friends who are engaged in this supreme act of love—helping one another to die for a justified, compassionate reason—have found it wise to work out an overtly declared pact explaining exactly what it is that the dying person requires.

In Holland, it is interesting to note, the Information Center for Voluntary Euthanasia (I.C.V.E.) provides people with a form letter which they can sign and place on their pillow after taking a lethal dose of drugs. This letter informs any person who is considering removing them to the hospital while they are in a coma, prior to death, that the unconscious person has specifically taken this action to end his or her own life after careful consideration because of a terminal illness; if this is doubted, advises the letter, one can telephone these friends (and the numbers are provided). The letter goes on to say that disturbing the comatose person would be an infringement of his or her civil rights to decline medical treatment, and the person will take subsequent civil court action against them if these rights are tampered with by resuscitation.

It is not against the law either to commit, or to attempt to commit, suicide (in most places). Therefore a successful civil suit could probably be brought against an unwanted revival of a dying person. In the U.S.A., the doctrine of *"informed* consent," which is well-defined in many court cases, would probably form an additional basis for the action, along with the traditional "battery"— medical treatment without consent.

The British voluntary euthanasia society, which was formed in 1935, recommends that people wanting to frustrate unwelcome interference with self-deliverance put a note beside them which reads as follows:

> *I have decided for the following reason to take my own life. This is a decision taken in a normal state of mind and is fully considered. (Give reasons.) I have the right not to be handled or treated against my will, and I absolutely forbid anyone to interfere with me while I continue to live. Anyone who disregards this notice will be committing a civil and criminal offense against me.*

An important guideline to doctors has been indicated in the medical magazine "The Lancet," (24 Jan., 1981), which stated in the context of an article discussing physician responsibilities to refer attempted suicide cases to psychiatrists (p. 196):

> *What should we aim to do for overdose patients in 1981? First, to recognize that an increasing number of rational individuals with no recognizable or treatable mental illness may wish to terminate their lives when their future seems likely to be irredeemably marred by physical or dementing disease. (The interest attracted by EXIT suggests that debates on euthanasia may be to the 1980s what our agonizing about abortion was to the 1960s.)*

Yet another tricky judgement to be made by a person intending self-deliverance is how long a period of time must be allowed for the ingested drugs to be certain to produce death? The thought of being revived is one which most horrifies euthanasists. Arranging prolonged privacy can take considerable planning.

The answer, of course, must lie chiefly with the lethality of the drugs used in each case. One hour is about the minimum with adequate barbiturates but death can take up to ten hours, depending on the dosage, body weight, how much already weakened by illness, other contents of the stomach, consumption of alcohol and so forth.

Based on the many cases related to me from different parts of the world, I consider that at least twelve hours of total seclusion must be ensured after an overdose has been taken. But with adequate overdosage, death ought to follow in an hour.

CHAPTER TEN

And we said nothing, all the day.

—JOHN DONNE

Discretion is indeed the watchword in an act of self-deliverance. The intention need not be kept a complete secret for, as the stories of Sonia Hertz and Jean Humphry showed, it has been found advisable to communicate the plan to one or two trusted confidants other than the person closest to the terminally ill individual (who should, in my view, always be told). Such communication can help if there are complications afterwards. Forewarned, it is easier to head off criticism or support the assister if he or she is under subsequent pressure from the authorities. All these decisions are, of course, entirely dependent on the personal circumstances of the terminally ill person, but certain guidelines are recommended.

After the death, it has always been found advisable for participants to maintain a cautious silence and let events run their course. (See appendix on law.) To make a verbal admission that one was even peripherally involved in a self-deliverance is to risk alerting the interest of a policeman or coroner who does not know the full circumstances, and is almost certainly unaware of the philosophy of the person recently deceased.

Carl Hertz shrewdly said nothing to arouse suspicions when the police and coroner's men came to his home at his request the morning Sonia died. "She's been very ill with cancer. She felt unwell this morning and went to bed. Then I found her dead," was the extent of the explanation he gave (or needed to give) to the authorities. When Jean died, my daughter-in-law telephoned the family doctor to ask him to come to certify death. As his car entered our driveway, I strolled out of the back door and took a walk in the fields until I saw him leave. Ruth Thomas, Margaret and Stella—the daughters of Mrs. Mercer—and Mary McFee (who had the most risk) all kept a discreet silence as far as the authorities were concerned. Subsequently they talked of their actions only to close friends as a necessary cartharsis for their grief.

Should a suicide note be left? It depends on the circumstances and must remain an individual judgement. On balance, I think it is prudent for the dying person considering self-deliverance to write a letter explaining the reasons for so doing and give this note to the closest friend who knows of the plan. The letter should only be produced if the legal authorities should happen to start proceedings.

The experience of one man in Palm Springs, California, who mentioned to the police his indirect involvement with his wife's suicide, is a cautionary tale.

The events happened in 1975; since then the man has moved to another part of the state and started a new life. Although the case was widely reported in the newspapers at the time, I will merely use his first name, Bill, because he prefers not to have attention drawn to himself today.

Bill's forty-nine-year-old wife, Francesca, suffered two years from a degenerative nervous disorder which affected the motor center of the brain and would have totally paralyzed her sooner or later. She was bedridden after five spinal operations and had lost the use of her left hand. After the fifth operation her doctors did not describe her as terminal, but they accepted that she would before long reach that state.

Francesca decided to end her suffering, so months beforehand she began taking fewer and fewer of her prescribed number of sleeping pills (Dalmane) and painkillers (Dilaudid)[32] until she considered that she had hoarded enough. During the next few weeks she dictated to her husband several letters for friends telling them that she did not expect to see them again. With some difficulty she signed her name at the bottom of the notes. She then dictated a final letter to her doctors, thanking them for increasing her medication and adding that she hoped she had been able to save enough pills to do the job well. She ended the letter with the words, "Goodbye, rotten world."

That evening Francesca called Bill into her room and said that she was tired of living in such an appalling manner and wanted to die. She then informed him that she had already taken two bottles of her pills. Soon afterwards she slipped into a coma, whereupon Bill propped her head up with a pillow and folded her arms, making her as comfortable as possible. For the next twenty-four hours he lovingly watched over her until she stopped breathing.

When he was certain that she was dead, he drew a sheet over her face and telephoned an ambulance. Francesca's illness and suicide had left him extremely despondent, and at that point he felt like committing suicide himself. In his distraction he told a young policeman who had accompanied the ambulance to the house: "I could not let her go on like this."

This remark alerted the officer, who started probing further. Bill then told him that he knew that his wife was planning suicide because of her illness, that he had agreed with her decision and that he had done nothing to stop it. Almost immediately the police arrested him for manslaughter. He was not kept in custody, however, but was released later that night on a $2,500 bond. The police chief said that the apparent omission of any preventive action by Bill made it a police responsibility, and it would be necessary to ask the district attorney if a criminal violation existed.

Bill then had to wait for six weeks before the district attorney made his decision

---

32. Dilaudid is a derivative of opium and is used to suppress the pain of terminal illness. Rated as "super toxic," the *Clinical Toxicology of Commercial Products* (Section II, p. 159) describes Dilaudid as "a more potent analgesic drug than morphine. Perhaps four times as toxic."

(in what lawyers agree is a grey area of the criminal law): there was to be no prosecution for any type of offense. Bill had not committed any crime because he had taken no direct actions, made no suggestions, and had merely agreed with his wife's self-deliverance—and not prevented it. Suicide is not a crime, so he could hardly be charged with conspiracy to commit something which was not a felony.

Looking back today, Bill says, "If I hadn't said anything, they wouldn't have known. Somehow I had to tell them; I was under such stress. I was so low, I didn't care what happened to me."

It has been the experience of most people involved with an act of self-deliverance from terminal illness that physicians, paramedics, ambulance crews, police and coroners will not normally delve into what has happened once they know that the deceased person was seriously ill. Such public servants see many sad cases of irrational suicide in the course of their week's work and generally have a sympathetic—if implicit—understanding of a sick person's rational suicide. They will not usually say so openly, and it is probably wisest not to put their loyalty and professionalism to the test by making an open admission of involvement. Such confessions may cause the official to feel obligated to mention the matters to his superiors. Then inevitably the chain of responsibility grows longer, more impersonal, and certainly more tortuous. In the end, even straightforward decisions can be extremely hard to resolve.

So long as an individual of his or her own free will has chosen to end life because a medical condition has made it unbearable, and so long as the person who assisted the suicide did so out of compassion (with no persuasion by either party), then the majority of people, authorities and otherwise, appear not to find either of these actions reprehensible. But it still remains prudent to bear in mind the old saying: "What the eye don't see, the heart don't grieve over."

A CHECKLIST

When you have read this book carefully, including the appendices, you will realise that active voluntary euthanasia (or suicide or self-deliverance, whatever you feel comfortable with calling it) is not a simple, easy matter. There is no way you can suddenly cut all ties with life, instantly disappear from the view of loved ones and friends, and, above all, the scientific preparations to be made require forethought and careful action.

Frequently the Hemlock Society receives complaints like "You've made it too complicated" and "Why can't I just go down to the hardware store, buy something, come home and take it and die quickly and painlessly?" The truth is that self-deliverance requires planning, patience and judgement.

The following is a summary of the main points already made in this little book which the terminally ill, mature adult should check over when contemplating their exit: -

1. Are you definitely dying? Make very sure. Get several opinions. Read medical news extensively to see if a cure is being developed.

2. When should it be done? We are only here once (or so I believe) and it is folly to leave too soon. Decide what is the criteria for an acceptable quality of life for *you*.

3. Can I wait until I am in the hospital for the last time? But how do you know when the last time is? Self-deliverance is nearly impossible in the hospital because of supervision; and is it fair to compromise the doctors and nurses?

4. Who will I hurt if I do this? It is advisable to tell those close to you what you are thinking. If they oppose you, tell them your philosophy and that *it is your life*. The reaction will probably be mixed. At least even those who have disagreed with you will not be shocked and surprised when you take your leave of this world.

5. Do I need help in securing privacy on my last day? Almost certainly yes. Find a sympathetic loved one who will either sit with you in your final sleep, or will at least stay outside and guard the door from interference.

6. Should I leave a written communication about my reasons for doing this? Probably yes. See previous chapter for advice and wording.

7. Make sure you have left a legal Will dealing with your estate. Your memory will be better respected if your financial affairs are tidy.

8. Should a "Living Will" be signed by me? Yes. They assist by giving a powerful indication of your views on dying and may even help in a legal dispute. (See back of book.)

9. If you are unfortunately obliged to end your life in a hotel, or somebody else's home, leave a note apologizing for the inconvenience caused. Explain the reasons briefly.

10. Leave instructions about how you wish your body to be disposed of— burial or cremation—and what type of service—in church or a memorial meeting—you desire.

11. Could there be a 'miracle cure' for my illness? If you sincerely believe so, then wait for one. Scientists will tell you that there is no such thing: medical progress is made in little steps forward, over years, and even the results need extensive testing.

12. If you are suffering unbearable physical pain, Hemlock urges two courses:

(A) Ask your physician for stronger pain killing drugs. Make your case to him as calmly and as factually as possible. Be persistent; if necessary see the physician's superior.

(B) If this way does not help, contact a Pain Control Center. Ask your physician to refer you, or find one yourself. Such centers are often attached to university medical centers. Use your telephone book or call your local library or newspaper.

Only a small percentage of terminal physical pain cannot be controlled today. As difficult as it sometimes is, there is no reason why you should suffer. There *is* help out there.

CHAPTER ELEVEN

How do I love thee? Let me count the ways.

—ELIZABETH BARRETT BROWNING

No one can truly say how they will cope with an act of voluntary euthanasia—either their own or a loved one's whom they may assist—until they actually face the experience. But it does help to think the matter through in advance. Some people on a philosophical level can decide in advance that they will accelerate the end of their lives if caught in a distressing illness; and some can decide that they will, if asked, help a loved one with the act of self-deliverance. On the other hand, some people decide in advance that they definitely will not seek euthanasia, preferring to battle it out to the end; others insist that under no circumstance could they assist another person to die, regardless of suffering and need.

In the years since I published *Jean's Way,* telling how I helped my own first wife to die, my 'confession' and the impact of the book, have induced many people to impart their innermost thoughts about dying to me. It has been my privilege to have been accorded a remarkable insight into their most private attitudes and prejudices on this sensitive subject. I have known those who swear they could never help their spouse die, although a rational request was made, but ultimately do provide the necessary aid and comfort, having resolved their inner conflicts and witnessed the increasing pain and anguish of their loved one. Yet there are others who positively agree to help in the self-deliverance of another and later have a change of heart.

There are those who decide on a carefully planned suicide to bring an end to their suffering, and have the courage and balance of mind to go through with it — even checking into a motel and taking an overdose, very privately, so that family members are not compromised legally or upset psychologically. I have known people who have helped loved ones or close friends to die and wanted to shout about it from the rooftops, feeling strongly that the law which they broke can only be changed by public testimony. (They usually take the advice of friends and end up being discreet.)

Some spouses insist upon sitting with their partner as they take their life with an overdose. A woman told me recently: "My husband had lung cancer for eight years, complicated with radiation side-effects, and made painful by emphysema. He got to the state where every breath was agony. When he decided to end his life, I wanted to sit with him, because we had loved each other for 30 years. I have no regrets at all that I was with him at the end." Another wife, who is a skilled nurse, told me how she had administered internally the fatal dose which killed her husband, a cancer sufferer. "We did it by agreement when he could take no more and knew that death was close," she said. "We had fought the disease together for three years; it seemed logical that the dying should be together and under our control."

It also happens that many self-proclaimed euthanasists often do not have the chance to conduct their self-deliverance (surely a more apt word in this context than suicide) because death comes to them too suddenly.

In the end, it all comes down to the character of the person and the individual circumstances of the particular dying experience. Factors that condition a person's attitude to voluntary euthanasia are frequently related to religious beliefs, which may be strong, moderate or completely lacking. Whether they were brought up to regard death as an integral part of life, or taught to shun it, and whether they believe in life after death also affects them. In some cases I have observed all these factors count for nothing: the clinching consideration is whether or not the person desiring an accelerated death, or the one asked to help, feels instinctively that it is right *for them*. This sense of "rightness" is based on a multitude of influences, the most important being the person's life experience.

In 1974, when Jean, my first wife, asked me to help her to die it came as a surprise since we had never previously discussed the matter. It did not strike me as a shocking option in view of her condition and nature. In fact, it seemed most sensible. She had bone cancer, with secondaries, and given her strong character, she had always demonstrated an ability to think things through calmly and to make decisions right for her.

I admired three things about her approach to her self-deliverance:

1. It was not to take place until we were convinced that no hope for further remission existed, and that no 'miracle' was on the horizon.

2. It was to be her decision alone, but to be guided by relevant information from me (such as observing whether she was acting out of depression or inner clarity.)

3. She had planned her death meticulously and was wholly unashamed of her intentions. In conversations with close friends, she would casually mention her plans.

When she first put the plan to me, I recall saying, instantly and intuitively, that if our positions were reversed and it was I who was dying, I would ask for the same help. Jean lived for another nine months after we made our pact. Those were rich and wonderful times for both of us. Though her body was crumbling from carcinomatosis, she was creative, loving and purposeful with every one, so much so that many could not believe she was dying, least of all that she knew it. Looking back I now believe it was her knowledge of the exact form death would take which gave her that peace of mind. It is an old truism that it is not death but the dying which is most frightening. Jean's home and family mirrored her life and achievements, and it was in that setting she wanted to depart. Given the nature of the disease she had contracted, she knew that if she did not take control of her dying, she would likely die in the corner of a hospital ward, probably in the middle of the night, having been virtually comatose for weeks from painkilling narcotics. She had spent too much time in cancer wards not to have witnessed many such deaths. It was this experience which strengthened her resolve to seek a more desirable end for herself.

As her death approached in the Spring of 1975, at the age of 42, I examined my conscience and the facts. I was about to be called on for my part of the bargain. Fortunately, we enjoyed intelligent, open communications with our medical advisors about Jean's condition, so there was no likelihood of a misunderstanding. She was very close to death. She had enjoyed her share of remissions, and any hope of a cure was — and still is — out of the question for her form of cancer.

Was it right to help? I reasoned that being asked by the person I loved most in the world, I could not refuse, even though it was a serious crime. (Suicide and attempted suicide are no longer crimes in the English-speaking world and many other countries, but assistance with suicide is still considered a crime and is sometimes punishable as murder.) I asked myself: doesn't love and long-term comradeship (we had been married 22 years) require that we stand by one another in time of dire need? I could not have lived with my conscience had I refused her plea to die, nor could I bear the thought that her attempted self-deliverance might be botched. Such a long and harrowing struggle for life (2½ years) deserved the reward of a good end on her own terms. I resolved to help, whatever the consequences. Since *Jean's Way* was published in 1978, it has had a mixed reception. Far more women than men are able to relate to the struggle which it outlines. I believe that women generally accept the reality of dying far more comfortably than men. My critics—and there are many— have called me 'murderer' and 'killer'. But I feel I did the right thing by Jean; their barbs have no effect. I am untroubled. Of course I did not 'kill' or 'murder' Jean. The ordinary connotation of those words is the taking of life without permission. What I did was to assist a rational person to end a life no longer tolerable.

After Jean's death, not one of the many persons who knew of my part in it chose to inform the police. The family doctor assumed cancer was the culprit and signed the death certificate. Three years later, when the book was published, there was considerable controversy; and the news media in Britain asked the police what they intended to do about my open confession of criminality. So the police were obliged to act. When the very gentlemanly senior detective arrived by appointment, I told him I was guilty of breaking the law, fully aware that it carried with it a penalty of up to 14 years imprisonment. I added that although I believed firmly in the rule of law (all my writings had born that out) Jean's death had been one of those rare and difficult occasions where personal conscience transcended law. If prosecuted, I would not contest the case, though I would argue strongly against a prison sentence. Ultimately the public prosecutor used his statutory discretion and did not charge me with any offense. One reason, I suppose, was that the 'crime' was then more than three years old and evidence would be difficult to marshal. Another reason for clemency, no doubt, was that substantial public opinion was demonstrably in favor of Jean's solution. Of course, the police also demanded the identity of the physician who had given me the lethal drugs. I refused to divulge it and they decided not to pursue the matter further. I certainly would not place this humane man's freedom and work in jeopardy on any account.

Most people involved in a euthanasia find no difficulty in putting the experience behind them. Many are proud of their act of love, so I find. And were I not at peace with myself, I could not agree to continual interviews on television and radio on the subject of Jean's death. I do not seek this exposure. Media people find Jean's tale a life-celebrating event worthy of the retelling more than once.

APPENDIX A

SOME SOCIAL ASPECTS OF TERMINAL ILLNESS

Background and Attitudes to the
Act of Self-Deliverance
by
Gerald A. Larue

Professor Emeritus of Biblical History and
Archaeology at the University of
Southern California, a Humanist
Counselor, and President of
the Hemlock Society

Active voluntary euthanasia as defined by Hemlock refers to any act to terminate life taken by someone who is in possession of his or her rational abilities after competent medical authorities have judged that person to be afflicted with an incurable disease and when that person experiences intractable pain as well as debasement of the human condition which robs life of dignity, meaning and purpose. Such acts of self-deliverance are commonly labelled "suicide." Despite the special conditions associated with these acts (such as unrelieved pain, paralysis, semi-comatose stupor, etc.) too often they come under the same kind of social and religious condemnation as any other act of suicide. For this and other reasons, we prefer to speak of active, rational, voluntary euthanasia as "self-deliverance" in the hope that the euphemism places some distance between the more irrational suicides and the very specific acts of life-taking that Hemlock is concerned with.

Attitudes Toward Suicide

Just what are these common attitudes toward suicide and where do they come from? For many, any act of self-killing automatically justifies condemnation. Typical labels such as "act of a coward," "over-reaction of a distrubed mind," "a sin against God," are used. In part, these reactions have grown out of our religious belief systems, in part out of society's uneasiness with an unnatural death, and in part out of personal feelings of dis-ease with any life-threatening phenomena.

Throughout history, every human society of which we have knowledge has developed rules and laws concerning the taking of life. Legislation prohibiting killing has always been designed to protect group members from lethal violence by other members and from life-threats from outside the group, but the patterns and the regulations have varied from community to community. For example, in some groups killing resulting from feuds and internecine struggles has

81

been accepted as "normal" and exempt from legal intervention or punishment, but not so in other groups. In many societies, killing in defence of one's own life or the lives of one's family and killing during war are usually categorized differently than ordinary murder. In other words, some forms of life-taking have been acceptable at certain times and under specific conditions.

When an individual ends his or her own life communal reactions can vary. In some societies the suicide is acceptable but only under certain conditions. Among some Esquimos when the aged reach a stage in life when they can no longer contribute to the welfare of the group, when they cannot enjoy their food and when the general quality of life is severely limited, they leave their igloo and go out into the Arctic to die by freezing. In Japan, prior to westernization of that culture, Harakiri was practiced by the warrior clan. Soldiers who were disgraced or who were sentenced to death disemboweled themselves in a ritual death. Among certain migratory tribes in Iran, the enfeebled still remain behind to die when the group makes its annual trek from the valleys to the mountains. A century ago in the British army, if an officer was discovered in some situation that "disgraced the uniform," he was permitted to "take the honorable way out" and shoot himself. None of these deaths were judged to be out of keeping with the standards of the cultures in which they existed.

In contemporary Western society, however, judgment is often passed on suicidal acts, whatever the reason. Sometimes the suicide has been termed "self-murder" and as such comes under the same disapproval as a killing. Although suicide is no longer against the law in any of the United States, society and religious disapproval so patterned over the ages still casts a bleak shadow over the lives of the family and friends of the dead person.

In broad terms, suicide has been called a crime against society because it robs the social group of human strength. What is perhaps more significant is that the act of self-killing symbolizes a challenge to traditional communal values which have been reinforced by theology, philosophy and common practice. The act defies traditional values; it raises questions about the meaning and value of life. It raises doubts about the idea that life must be preserved at all costs— no matter how its quality and significance may have been eroded by debilitating and dehumanizing illness. For some, suicide disturbs the tranquility of accepted mores, beliefs and attitudes.

Because suicide has been viewed as a cowardly or emotionally disturbed act, it is perceived of as an anomaly. "He went round the bend," of "She just snapped," are typical comments. Such interpretations imply that there must have been some abnormal dimension to the suicide's life, some mental or emotional aberration to provoke non-normal behavior. In no way can such viewers understand rational suicide. The negative labelling reflects the ubiquitous uneasiness society feels toward any act of self-killing. The implication is that a normal, well-adjusted, rational individual would never kill himself, regardless of life's pressures.

In general, suicide has been judged a crime against God and considered a sin because, according to some theology, the deity gave life and only the deity should determine when life ends. Yet, interestingly enough, suicide appears to have been accepted in the religions of many ancient societies. For example, suicide is not specifically condemned or prohibited in the Bible, unless the commandment "Thou shalt not kill" (which is correctly translated "You shall not commit homicide") be interpreted to include suicide. King Saul and his armor-bearer committed suicide rather than fall into the hands of the enemy Philistines (I Sam. 31:4-5; I Chron. 10:4-5). There was no condemnation. Nor was King Zimri of Israel faulted when he died in a fire he himself had ignited at a time of desperation (I Kings 16:15-20). When Ahitophel, King David's counselor, hanged himself there was no denouncement of him and he was buried in his family tomb (II Sam. 17:23). Nor was Judas condemned when he hanged himself (Matt. 27:5).

Despite the lack of condemnation of suicide in the Bible, the early Christian church did move away from it as an acceptable way to end life. St. Augustine (A.D. 354-430) condemned suicide as a violation of the *sixth* commandment. Later, St. Thomas Aquinas (1225-1274) argued that the act was a mortal sin: he declared that it was contrary to natural law, damaging to the human community, and symbolic of humans usurping divine prerogatives concerning decisions of life and death. Such attitudes have become the heritage of the Christian Church and particularly the Roman Catholic Church—and hence of society in general.

Traditionally, Roman Catholic clergy have refused funeral rites and burial in consecrated grounds to suicide victims. Church cemeteries had separated areas of interment for anyone who had died without the blessings of the church. Fenced off from sacred grounds (and often untended and overgrown with weeds), these graves became stark reminders of the church's rejection of anyone who violated religious taboos.

In recent years, however, there has been a change. Many Catholic priests do not refuse church rites nor burial in Roman Catholic cemeteries to victims of suicide. These priests acknowledge that social forces and the complex pressures of modern existence often confuse and disorient individuals. It becomes impossible to fix responsibility and blame solely upon the victim; society is also accountable.

Protestant and Jewish clergy also tend to treat the issue of suicide with compassion and understanding. For those who belong to Ethical Culture and Humanist groups, suicide is viewed as one way of terminating life and there is no condemnation of the individual. No guilt is fixed on the friends and family of the deceased person. On the other hand, suicide is prohibited among Muslims as a violation of the divine will and the teachings of the Quran. Those who take their own lives are excluded from the Muslim paradise.

Among philosophers, suicide has often been regarded as an acceptable way to end life despite the religious taboos. For example, the utilitarian philosopher David Hume (1711-1776) could find no valid argument against suicide—neither legal nor moral nor religious. The existentialist philosopher, Albert Camus

(1914-1960) proposed suicide as a logical way to resolve the absurdity of life. As we have noted, members of Ethical Culture groups and the American Humanist Association attach no guilt or blame to suicide. Indeed, the Humanist Manifesto II published in 1973 states:

> To enhance freedom and dignity the individual must experience a full range of civil liberties in all societies. This includes freedom of speech and the press, political democracy, the legal right of opposition to governmental policies, fair judicial process, religious liberty, freedom of association, and artistic, scientific, and cultural freedom. *It also includes a recognition of an individual's right to die with dignity, euthanasia, and the right to suicide.* (Italics mine)

There have, of course, been some who have warned that if suicide is accepted as a human right, it will be easily abused. It has been said that those who have contemplated taking their own lives in the past—but who hesitated because of moral, ethical, religious and social pressures—will be encouraged to do so. Perhaps there is some truth to this argument, but on the other hand, for the terminally ill, arguments based on moral, religious, social or any other groups can be irrelevant. Furthermore, suicide, once it has happened, is really neither right nor wrong. It is simply an act. Judgement must be in the minds of those who live on, and such judgement is usually based on highly subjective criteria which can be questioned and challenged.

Consideration of active voluntary euthanasia by the terminally ill is a personal statement. It is a statement made when life has lost its significance and is no longer worth living. The unendurable is there: illness, weakness, pain, negative prognoses, no prospects of cure or remission, and no easing of the suffering—all of which rob one's existence of joy and pleasure. The all-important *now* is burdened with efforts to cope and little or no relief. To exist is wearisome and draining. Pain and mind-deadening drugs reduce life to mere survival in an uncomfortable, stupor-like state. It may be time for release; it may be time to accept the advantages and benefits of rational, voluntary euthanasia.

The word "euthanasia," derived from two Greek terms *eu* meaning "good" and *thanatos* meaning "death," can be interpreted as signifying "a good death" or "a beneficial death" or an "acceptable death." Sometimes one hears the phrase "mercy killing" for euthanasia, but this is not a satisfactory substitute. "Killing" by definition implies the taking of a life against the will of the person who is to die, or has died. Clearly this is not the same as euthanasia, although the two are often confused. Unfortunately the terms have been further muddled by their association with the Nazis during World War II to describe the extermination of people whom the Nazis found unacceptable. As we have noted, although Hemlock continues to use the word euthanasia, there is a distinct preference for the term self-deliverance.

In the popular press, one reads of two kinds of euthanasia: passive and active. Passive euthanasia refers to the absence of "heroic measures" to sustain the life of a dying person. In other words, when a patient is being kept alive by mechanical means—when there is no hope that he or she will be able to live without the machine and when the future promises to be burdened by further pain and coma—the life-support systems are removed and the individual is permitted a "natural" death. Of course, death is not always instantaneous and sometimes the period of life after removal of the support equipment is marked with distressing responses.

The most famous case of "passive euthanasia" in the United States is that of Karen Ann Quinlan who lapsed into a coma on April 14, 1975. On May 17, 1976, after a lengthy court battle, Karen was removed from the respirator. She is still alive in 1981—a comatose eighty-pound figure, curled in a fetal position and kept alive by intravenous feeding. She is completely unaware of the outside world and completely dependent upon others for existence. One cannot consider this and similar cases without raising some questions about the value and quality of life, about human dignity, and about what such insistence on the maintaining of life at this level says about our society.

Most religious organizations support the passive euthanasia concept. There are still some groups that insist that "Only God gives life and only God should take it away," and that medical science should make every effort to keep life going until God makes the decision. However, these groups are in a minority. Contemporary Judeo-Christian thinking now sanctions and accepts the principle of passive euthanasia.

In December 1973, the American Medical Association adopted a "death with dignity" report urging doctors to respect a dying patient's wishes regarding the amount of medical care they were to receive. Yet decisions to remove life-support systems still come hard to many medical doctors—they are, after all, committed to healing and restoring a person to health, not to ending life. Some are concerned about legal problems, and rightly so. To help avoid litigation, a directive to physicians called "The Living will" has been produced by the Euthanasia Education Council (now known as "Concern for Dying") and is available to anyone who requests a copy. In some states such as California, bills have been passed permitting terminally ill patients to order an end to artificial life-sustaining procedures. Such documents are designed both to protect the physician from prosecution and to place the patient in control of his or her own death.

The issue of "active euthanasia," taking positive steps to end the life of the terminally ill—is a major concern of Hemlock. As we have stated many times, our concern is with the terminally or incurably ill who have made *rational* decisions about ending their own life. Although there has been no widespread acceptance of active voluntary euthanasia, Hemlock has received hundreds of letters which suggest that this once-tabooed, hidden and suppressed issue of self-deliverance is beginning to surface and will continue to become a significant issue in discussions of medical ethics and human values. As this book demonstrates, there are numerous cases in which terminally ill individuals have attempted and succeeded in delivering themselves from pain and suffering— sometimes acting alone, but often supported and aided by caring, loving friends and relatives.

We are only now beginning to grapple with some of the problems arising from the use of advanced technology developed by modern medical and engineering sciences for prolonging life. In many, indeed, in most situations the equipment is used effectively and positively, and patients, families and medical practitioners can only be grateful for the advances. But there are some unique circumstances in which keeping an individual alive become questionable. When the significance of life has decayed and the experience of pain is unremitting, it is time to question the purpose of such life-sustaining equipment and the failure to use lethal drugs to end the suffering of an already-dying person. One asks: which is the greater expression of love and caring—to maintain life by whatever means (and cost) despite the patient's wish to die and the knowledge that the patient's life has been reduced to a less-than-human level, or to deliver that person from further suffering and degradation? For members of the Hemlock Society the answer appears to be clear; for others it is indeed a shadowy ethical problem.

So far, there has been no in-depth response from religious organizations to Hemlock. A few letters have expressed indignation on the rather traditional grounds that we have previously noted. Perhaps because we focus on individuals who are in the final stages of life and who are in pain, and who also wish to take charge of their own deliverance, can our form of suicide be considered acceptable. Then again, perhaps religious organizations have not yet become fully aware of all the implications in our proposals and find the issue of self-deliverance to be peripheral. Only time will tell.

No one should feel compelled to confront self-deliverance alone. Hardly anyone feels more separated, more isolated and more abandoned than the terminally ill when they decide that they no longer want to live. Numerous Hemlock members have written to us about their feelings and about the impossibility of communicating their wishes and intentions to loved ones or friends. When they introduce the subject, too often their statements are dismissed, their feelings are denied, and their efforts to share are blocked. They are convinced that family and friends not only cannot understand what they feel, but may indeed take steps to prevent an act of self-deliverance.

Despite the conspiracy of silence, there are a number of reasons why intentions and wishes should be shared with friends and relatives. Because self-deliverance is technically a suicidal act, those who remain to mourn may grieve with an additional burden of guilt because of their lack of communication with the deceased person. They may feel that they are excluded from the most private and meaningful intentions of someone they loved and that they failed in their love and friendship. They are bound to feel that they were inadequate companions. Regrets take the form of "I wish I had told her..." "I ought to have listened to him or paid attention to him..." "If only I could have..." In each instance a conflict is represented between what was done (or not done) and what should have been done. The effect is both guilt-producing and anxiety-producing.

Yet the initial barriers in communicating are easy to understand. It is possible to be put off by the protestations of those we love most or by their efforts to divert conversation from what we wish to convey, expecially when the subject is as painful as impending death. We in turn become protective of their feelings and hesitate to assert our own needs lest we upset or offend. In short, people close to the terminally ill person can engage in a form of denial by blocking attempts to initiate conversation about the termination of life. Responding to this "cue," the patient inadvertently reinforces the distance by avoiding a touchy subject. Because of the intricate—and often subliminal—network of communication it is important to understand another's basic fear of death. On broader levels, society engenders patterns of denial by classifying conversations about death as socially unacceptable and taboo. To talk about death is to put someone in touch with his or her own mortality, and for many this results in most uncomfortable feelings. It is easier to avoid the subject altogether.

Perhaps it is possible to introduce discussion on the subject while at the same time respecting the wishes of our friends and family to avoid feelings of fear and discomfort. Wait for the moment when you are clear in your thinking and your mind is not too clouded by drugs and your pain is not too severe. It is important to be firm and direct. "I have something I want to share with you. you may not like what I will say, but it is important that I say it. Please hear me without interruption..."

Once an agreement to listen has been reached, you can control the tendency to interrupt by simply raising your hand in a gesture that signals "Please wait." Then communicate as clearly and as briefly as you can what you intend to do. If your hearer (or hearers) wishes to argue with you, listen to what you are being told. Understand their feelings of anger and dismay and discomfort, but do not engage in argument. There is no reason that everyone must agree with you, and there is no reason that you must agree with others. There may be tears and other signs of emotional upset, but these are responses of caring people who are confronting loss. Sometimes it becomes necessary to ask over and over again for a hearing and for permission to speak. But once heard, one can begin to make plans for the ending of life including arranging for special opportunities to convey feelings of love and caring, making plans for the distribution of personal items, reaching out to those who matter most, talking about the past, and giving help to those who will remain to cope with the future.

Needless to say, a tremendous burden rests upon those of you who take responsibility for your own death. You leave survivors who must grapple with feelings of loss, emptiness, grief and guilt. Early sharing enables you and those you care about to begin the grieving process early. You grieve over the anticipated separation and about the brevity of human life; they grieve as they anticipate life without you.

Some who are at present in good health are making public statements about what should happen to them in case of a debilitating accident or illness which will lead to an early death. They have communicated to their friends and loved ones what they want to have done—and *not* done to them. Because they are in good health, the possibility of such a situation may seem remote, but such sharing becomes a kind of insurance against total helplessness in the face of a protracted deathbed. Some make verbal agreements with family members, and others share their wishes with doctors and lawyers. These decisions, made when the individual is rational and healthy, help to ease the difficulty of introducing dialogue about self-deliverance during a painful, terminal illness when all too often their judgment will be distrusted.

It may seem unfair to involve someone else in one's decision to end life. Certainly there are those who feel anger when they are included. On the other hand, the trauma experienced by those who feel they were excluded after a loved one's death appears to be more devastating than the anger.

As we have learned from the accounts recorded in this and from our legal counsel, there is some peril in involving others in one's death. They may be charged with aiding and abetting a suicide and be subject to prosecution. None of us wants that to happen to someone we care about. But, as we have seen, there are situations when the ill person clearly needs assistance. At present there seems to be no way to handle this problem easily. Each individual must decide for herself or himself to what degree he or she will become involved. Each individual must determine the extent of his own commitment and the risks involved. Is involvement worth the risk? Is non-involvement worth the guilt?

One of the saddest comments I heard was at an international conference of right-to-die societies; a man who failed to help a friend to die reflected on his guilt. "I've carried the burden of my indecision ever since then," he commented sadly. On the other hand, there may be those who have aided in an act of self-deliverance and regretted their actions. So far we have not heard from any of these. We do know, however, of those who have provided assistance and who have been penalized.

There are some medically-trained people who will help; there are more who will not. One acquaintance of mine has three sons, each of whom is a doctor. He has promises from each that should the time come when he is terminally ill and wishes to take his own life but is too weak or helpless to do so, they will help him. Not many are so fortunate or privileged as he.

We are learning that the more we open up the subject of active voluntary euthanasia, the closer we move to the time when we and our loved ones will be protected by law should self-deliverance become an issue. We are approaching the time when doctors and lawyers, ethicists, clergy and concerned groups will have to consider legislation to protect one's right to self-deliverance.

From accounts of those who have participated in acts of self-deliverance—

relatives of the now deceased and diaries and letters of the terminally ill— we learn of feelings which are almost euphoric. These people have come to terms with dying. They no longer fear death. Anyone who has assisted someone else to die with dignity knows that he has acted out of love and that he has confronted and overcome a fear of dying. These people talk of feelings that defy description. One man who survived a life-death crisis spoke of feelings as if he had died and that death will never again burden him; he can now face whatever will be his final moment with calmness. His exuberance is not that of wild, leaping joy, but of quiet excitement in life and acceptance of himself as the person in control.

Feelings of tranquility, control or joy, however, do not eliminate grieving or mourning. Indeed there are those who have participated in a loved one's self-deliverance and who feel comfortable about their involvement, but who still feel pain and deep emotion when they recall their association with the loved person. To participate voluntarily in the death of another is not to render one immune to the emotional responses of caring and grief. Nor does one become callous and insensitive. On the contrary, such people seem to be among the most caring, the most gentle, the most involved and the most committed of individuals. There can be little doubt that their participation in death has brought a mellowing dimension to their existence.

Closing a Relationship

The term "closure" refers to the sealing of relationships, the healing of wounds, the settling of differences, the salving of irritations, the bonding of individuals and the closing of gaps in human relating. Perhaps the most difficult problem to deal with in grief therapy occurs when the living have failed to achieve closure with those who have died. Words that were never spoken, feelings that were never expressed, apologies that were never given seem to hover over them like incompleted sentences. The guilt is daunting: guilt over unresolved differences, over failures to express more love and concern and over hesitation to utter words of appreciation and love can haunt the living.

Closure is not something that needs to be put off until the time of dying; it is a process to be engaged in at all times. We live in a happenstance world. Death can come at any moment by accident, violence, natural disaster or a sudden failure of some essential organ to function properly. We cannot count on living to a ripe old age and then dying quietly in the presence of our loved ones having made closure with each. We can die at any time and therefore it is important to continually seek to make closure with those whom we love. Closure involves expressing our love and caring when we separate for longer or shorter times. Closure means settling our differences as rapidly as possible and not letting old wounds fester. It is not necessary to wait until plans for self-deliverance are being discussed with someone terminally ill. Closure is a daily responsibility. And when one is terminally ill, it is of vital importance that gaps in relationships be reduced and love expressed.

How is this done? For some it is very difficult. Many families have developed patterns of reticence in communicating deep feelings. They do not say "I love you"; they assume that others know, somehow, that they are loved. A thirty-two-year-old daughter told me that only as her mother lay in a terminal coma was she able to speak to the inert figure and pour out her feelings of love. Could the mother hear her? As she spoke about her love and concern, the fingers of the comatose woman tightened on her hand. I assured the young woman that her mother had heard and had responded. We now know that individuals who are by all medical standards unconscious of the world about them (if they have not suffered brain damage) do hear and are not completely insensitive to the world about them. But how tragic to have waited so long! And how fortunate and how healing to know that there was a response!

A woman who had not achieved closure with a daughter who had taken her own life was haunted by hallucinatory experiences in which her daughter appeared and seemed to be requesting her mother to join her in death. Of course the images were products of the mother's mind and grew out of her feelings of lack of closure. Through image therapy the gap was eventually closed.

Meaningful relationships must be worked at. Part of the procedure involves achieving closure regularly. Where closure has been made, grief and the grieving process are made infinitely easier.

Grief and Grieving

Death produces feelings of separation, loss, emptiness and sometimes abandonment. The processes of grief and grieving involve coping with those feelings.

There is no proper or correct way to grieve. Among some the expressions are open, free, unrestricted and perhaps even noisy. With others, grief is quieter and turned inward rather than outward. Grief can continue for long or short periods of time and may produce reactions of deep sadness and even physical pain. Memories flood the mind and bring tears. Small tokens associated with the dead provoke long past associations and elicit warm although painful recollections. All of these are healthy reminders of our humanity.

When grief and the grieving process begin to produce "toxic" responses, those who are closest to the mourner may be properly concerned. Toxic grief is grief that will not release the dead. The person continues to function as though the dead person were still part of the world of the living. Decisions are made according to what it is believed the dead person would have wanted. Furniture must be kept in the same positions as the deceased arranged it. The survivor begins to withdraw from the world of the living, performing only the basic associations necessary for survival, but focusing more and more on the past and on the deceased. When meals are not eaten and health is neglected, there is genuine cause for concern. Both medical help and therapeutic counseling are called for.

Nourishing grief does not deny the significance of the dead person, nor does it turn away from mourning processes or ignore memories. It *does* turn the griever back to the world of the living. It helps to develop out of crisis situations new potentials for meaning-filled living. It recognizes that life must go on. It helps the individual accept life one day at a time until the deepest feelings of hurt and loss and pain are somewhat alleviated and the mind can constructively carry on with life without the dead person.

The presence of caring persons is most important during this time and friends can help the mourning person most by encouraging the griever to express the myriad of emotions that are there. Perhaps the most helpful question one can ask is, "Will you tell me what happened?" Each time the story is told, grief will come, but each time the compassionate listener gives the mourner permission to grieve. The more often the story is told, the better. Each telling is an airing of feelings.

On some occasions grief will be tempered by feelings of relief. The pain and the suffering are ended; the ailing person has been released, and the struggle with the dying process is over. If closure has been made and if the death has come in an acceptable way, it is normal to feel that an episode or a segment of living has been completed. It is time to take a deep breath and look again to the world of the living; it is time to give energy to nourishing the self and those who remain. A good and acceptable death releases not only the terminally ill, but also those who have waited and watched, cared and cried, reached out and were in turn responded to, hoped and felt hope ebb. The ordeal is over. The end has come. It is time for a new beginning.

APPENDIX B

The legal background to suicide and assisted suicide

by

Curt Garbesi

Professor of Law, Loyola Law School, Los Angeles.
Legal consultant to the Hemlock Society.

The history of suicide law is a barbaric tale. Not only did our forebears make it a felony to commit suicide, their law required mutilation of the body and burial in disgrace. Further, all property was forfeited to the King, adding to the misery and mental anguish of family and friends. Not so very long ago, even in the United States, suicide was considered "self murder"—although confiscation of goods was never part of our law as it was in some countries; and the deceased was, of course, beyond the power of punishment by the State. Attempted suicide which failed, however, was a punishable crime—providing doubtlessly unintended inducement to success.

It is now generally established that neither an attempted nor a successful act of self-deliverance entails penal liability—although it may have some legal effect. Today, the law comes to bear on those considered "accomplices" to the act. Thus, it is with the issue of their liability that I am dealing here.

The right to free speech is protected under the United States constitution. A little reflection would suggest, however, that even so basic a right must have some limitations. Most of us probably would agree with an illustrious nineteenth century Supreme Court jurist that no one should be entitled to shout "FIRE!" in a crowded theatre unless there really is a fire. Nor would we disagree with prohibitions upon disclosure of atomic weaponry secrets to terrorist groups. The problem lies in drawing the line between protected verbal conduct and that which is legitimately subject to control.

Society has perhaps as much interest in protecting life as it does in assuring freedom to exchange ideas. When either conflicts with the other, it is necessary to decide which must give way. Basically, our law clearly protects general discussions on any subject, including those concerning termination of life. If this results in someone's being better informed, and therefore able to commit suicide, this is a risk we accept for the benefits of free intercourse. So, anyone should feel free to discuss such matters openly, and even to advocate particular, carefully detailed techniques for self-deliverance. But, when a discussion of generalities becomes advocacy of individual action, the conduct may be punishable. Such advocacy is characterized as "solicitation".

The Penal Law

Solicitation

Many states punish the mere solicitation of another to commit a crime. Dependent on the niceties of local law, simple encouragement of another to end his own life also may be criminally punishable. And, to further complicate matters, the line between general discussion and the advocacy of individual action is not always easy to discern. In the gray area, police and prosecutors may decide to prefer charges, and let a court decide whether it was a crime. Anyone who has experience with courts and lawyers knows he should strive mightily to avoid such entaglement. One way is to avoid reference to individuals who need help, let alone any conduct or statements that might be interpreted as giving encouragement to an individual to end his or her life.

Conspiracy

If two or more people join together to commit a crime, to do a wrong to another, or even to do something as ambiguously defined as "subverting public morals," they can be convicted of a serious crime. This does not mean that a group who discuss crime in general, or even discuss quite specific means of committing a particular criminal act transgress. However, once the conversation shifts into planning for a definite goal which is prohibited by the law, the conduct becomes severely punishable. Here, too, the dividing line between the legitimate and the criminal is highly cloudy; so, be cautious.

In addition to the crime of conspiracy itself, i.e., the planning of specific prohibited conduct, each of those who engages in it is responsible for any crime committed by a co-conspirator, which is a natural outcome of their joint conspiracy. This is the case, even if the specific crime was not planned or even contemplated by the group. For example, if the conduct of any one conspirator can be found to have contributed to causing a death (e.g., providing the instrument or even simple encouragement of the death-causing act), then, however humane the objective, all face the possibility of serious penalties.

Avoidance of such risks requires that no group come to an understanding, whether explicit or tacit, that any one of them will encourage another (even another member of the group) to take his or her own life. Should a death occur, which could be traced in part to the conspiracy, then each and every member of the group could conceivably be prosecuted and convicted of criminal homicide.

An important subsidiary point in the law of conspiracy is that the parties charged need not ever have met together or even conversed with one another in order to be open to criminal prosecution. A case in point is the euthanasia support groups. For instance, it is sufficient to establish that all those charged with the crime consciously sought the same illegal goal in support of each other. Not even the identity of the other group members need be known to each defendant.

The next question is, what kind of conduct is punishable because it somehow contributes to the suicide of another? I have already discussed solicitation to commit the act. And in some jurisdictions, the term "solicitation" is not limited to verbal solicitation. That is to say—any conduct which is intended to or which tends to encourage the suicide of another is sufficient grounds for legal prosecution. The range of "aiding and abetting" may be extended to include a "failure to protect". For instance, a father who stands by and passively watches his child swallow poison—which both of them know is intended to cause death—would be guilty of aiding and abetting the act.

Even in those jurisdictions where solicitation of a suicide is not considered criminal independent of results, if the solicitee attempts suicide, the solicitor could be charged with anything from "criminal solicitation" to "battery" to "attempted manslaughter". And, if the attempt were successful, he could conceivably be convicted of murder.

If mere solicitation can have such profound implications, then acts of aiding and abetting leave one wide open to prosecution. The most obvious among these would be the actual administration of a lethal dose. Short of that, providing the poison or other means of death—with the intent to help cause that death—is also criminal. Placing poison within reach would suffice. It must be emphasized throughout that liability to punishment is not dependent on proof of an evil motive, nor is proof of a beneficent one a defense. All that need be established is the intent to act in such a way as to aid or abet an act resulting in death. Depending on the outcome, charges could be brought for criminal solicitation, attempted murder, or murder itself.

Civil Law Problems

Licensing

Pharmacists and medical practitioners—among some other kinds of professionals—must be licensed in order to function legally within their professions. A student in one of these disciplines who used his or her knowledge to aid in a suicide might be denied a license. Once a person is licensed to practice in a particular profession, evidence of professional misconduct might well result in license suspension or revocation. That explains the natural reticence on the part of health care professionals to aid suicides; and it is exceedingly difficult to get aid from that quarter.

In the case of physicians, the problem is even more acute, since the question of continued hospital staff membership may be in jeopardy. Even if the risk is relativeley minor that revocation of privileges actually would occur, it is an additional consideration reducing the probability of aid just that much more.

Most life insurance policies include clauses making them inoperative if the insured dies of suicide within two years of the policy's issuance. This reduces the risk of someone's taking out a policy for the purpose of conferring a substantial benefit on a loved one by shortly ending his own life. But, if the suicide takes place *after* two years, the benefits generally must be paid, according to local law.

Double indemnity clauses (double payment) are brought into effect by accidental deaths, not intentional ones. Thus, at any time after the suicide limitation period, if the insurance company can establish that what appeared to be an accident was in fact a suicide, it will only be responsible for basic coverage.

Similarly with estates, the beneficiary of a life insurance policy who is convicted of murdering the insured may not benefit from the policy. The proceeds normally are then paid into the estate. Thus, a beneficiary who encourages or assists in the suicide of the insured risks losing not only his freedom, but also his insurance benefits.

Estates

Those whose aid is most frequently sought by a would-be suicide are close relatives or friends. They are also the most likely to be beneficiaries of the estate, whether by will or by operation of law. In the event that a person, who otherwise would take from the estate, should be convicted of murder (or possibly a less serious criminal homicide) of the deceased, the law, in many states, precludes his sharing in a subsequent distribution. This is consistent with the common law principle that "one should not profit from his own wrong." Although we may well question whether it is a moral "wrong" to aid in a suicide, the principle is applied rigorously in all cases of conviction, regardless of mitigating circumstances.

Civil Liability

In the area of civil liability for damages, it is well established that one who has committed a crime, including conspiracy against another, may be held responsible for damages as well.

Even short of criminal conduct, one who intentionally or negligently causes injury or death to another is also subject to liability for damages at the behest of the injured party or, in case of death, his survivors or estate. There are two possible scenarios to be examined: the botched suicide attempt and the successful one.

If a person "negligently" assists another in an unsuccessful attempt to take his own life, no remedy would be available merely on the basis of failure. Failure to succeed in conduct conceived of as criminal or "wrongful" cannot be the basis of recovery. Since the death is not thought to be desirable legally, one has a duty to avoid causing it, regardless of the wishes of the target. Thus the unintended result of the "negligence" coincides with what the law would dictate; and no court would predicate liability upon it. However, the conduct in question might have aggravated a pre-existing condition, causing greater pain and expense; or, it could have caused some new injury. In either case, liability could ensue.

If the subject were incompetent at the time of the attempt, the assister clearly would be liable for all damage caused by it. (This would not include the ordinary costs of continued living not affected adversely by the attempt.) However if the subject is in control of his or her faculties, it is probable that causation and contributory fault theory would reduce or entirely avoid liability. Assuming that the subject is equally capable of appreciating the risks inherent in his or her conduct—and of avoiding them—he or she should be held at least equally responsible for them. Of course, if the assister either had or purported to have special expertise (e.g., to be a doctor, nurse or other health care professional) then a substantial percentage of the damage could be attributed to him or her.

It is fair to assume that any liability for failed assistance would probably be relatively minor. Since the would-be suicide's life was likely to be of limited duration, the likelihood of very substantial damages being awarded is relatively slight.

In cases of successful aided suicides, there is the possibility of the assister being held liable to survivors for causing the death. All jurisdictions have laws which permit recovery from one who wrongfully causes the death of another. The same arguments of causation and contributing fault of the deceased, mentioned in the preceding paragraphs, are applicable here. However, the substantial probability of some liability cannot be excluded.

Since the "value" to others of the continued existence of one so ill that suicide was the solution is undoubtedly small, substantial damages are not likely in any wrongful death action. However, it is nonetheless desirable to avoid the probability of suit, if that is at all possible. One way to reduce the likelihood of suit and recovery is to get the concurrence of immediate family members in the self-deliverance plans. If they are themselves involved, they are much less likely to complain, and their probability of success is that much more improbable.

Conclusion

Anyone who contemplates suicide or assisting another to do so should be well aware of the risks involved. The Hemlock Society, its officers and directors, do not advocate suicide under any circumstances. However, they do advocate the right of each person to make that ultimate choice, and of others to assist in carefully defined circumstances. We hope one day to be able to rewrite this section to reflect changes brought about by our efforts to liberalize the law. With your support, we feel we can and will succeed.

STATES HAVING SPECIFIC PENAL LAWS REGARDING ASSISTING SUICIDE

ASKA

Manslaughter...(2) intentionally aids another person to commit suicide. (AS, Section 11.41.120)

IZONA

A person commits manslaughter by:

...intentionally aiding another to commit suicide. (ARS, Section 13-1103)

LIFORNIA

Every person who deliberately aids, or advises, or encourages another to commit suicide, is guilty of a felony. (Penal Code, Section 401)

NNECTICUT

A person is guilty of manslaughter in the second degree when:

...he intentionally causes or aids another person, other than by force, duress or deception, to commit suicide. (Penal Code, Section 53a-56)

AWARE

A person is guilty of promoting suicide when he intentionally causes or aids another person to attempt suicide, or when he intentionally aids another person to commit suicide.

Promoting suicide is a ...felony. (11 Del C Section 645)

RIDA

Every person deliberately assisting another in the commission of self-murder shall be guilty of manslaughter, a felony of the second degree, punishable as provided in sections...(Florida Statutes, Section 782.08)

WAII

A person commits the offense of manslaughter if:

...he intentionally causes another person to commit suicide. (HRS, Section 707-702)

IANA

a person who intentionally causes another human being, by force, duress, or deception, to commit suicide commits causing suicide, a ...felony. (IC, Section 35-42-1-2.)

ISAS

Assisting suicide is intentionally advising, encouraging or assisting another in the taking of his own life.

Assisting suicide is a ...felony. (KSA, 21-3406.)

NE

A person is guilty of aiding or soliciting suicide if he intentionally aids or solicits another to commit suicide, and the other commits or attempts suicide. Aiding or soliciting suicide is a ...crime. (17-A MSRA, Section 204.)

NESOTA

Whoever intentionally advises, encourages, or assists another in taking his

own life may be sentenced to imprisonment for not more than 15 year
or to payment of a fine of not more than $15,000, or both. (Criminal Code
Section 609.215.)

MISSISSIPPI

A person who willfully, or in any manner, advises, encourages, abets, o
assists another person to take, or in taking, the latter's life, or in attemp
ting to take the latter's life, is guilty of felony and, on conviction, sha
be punished by imprisonment in the penitentiary not exceeding ten years
or by fine not exceeding one thousand dollars, and imprisonment in th
county jail not exceeding one year. (Miss. Code, Section 97-3-49

MONTANA

A person who purposely aids or solicits another to commit suicide, bu
such suicide does not occur, commits the offense of aiding or solicitin
suicide.

A person convicted of the offense of aiding or soliciting a suicide shall b
imprisoned in the state prison for any term not to exceed 10 years,or b
fined an amount not to exceed $50,000 or both. (RCM, Section 45-5-105

NEBRASKA

A person commits assisting suicide when, with intent to assist another per
son in commiting suicide, he aids and abets him in commiting or attemp
ting to commit suicide. Assisting suicide is a class IV felony. (Neb. RS
Section 28-307)

NEW HAMPSHIRE

A person is guilty of causing or aiding suicide if he purposely aids or solicit
another to commit suicide.

Causing or aiding suicide is a ...felony if the actor's conduct causes suc
suicide or an attempted suicide. Otherwise it is a misdemeanor. (RSA, Sec
tion 630:4.)

NEW JERSEY

(Common law offense indictable as misdemeanor, if suicide is committed
(New Jersey Statutes 2A:85-1; 2A:85-14)

NEW MEXICO

Assisting suicide consists of deliberately aiding another in the taking of hi
own life. Whoever commits assisting suicide is guilty of a ...felony. (NMSA
30-2-4.)

NEW YORK

A person is guilty of murder in the second degree when:
...the defendant's conduct consisted of causing or aiding, without the us
of duress or deception, another person to commit suicide. (New York Pena
Law, Section 125.25 (b))

OKLAHOMA

Every person who willfully in any manner advises, encourages, abets c
assists another person in taking his own life is guilty of aiding suicide. (Okla
Stat. tit. 21, Section 813) Every person guilty of aiding an attempt at suicid

is punishable by imprisonment in the penitentiary not exceeding two years, or by a fine not exceeding $1,000, or both. (Okla. Stat. tit. 21, Section 818)

OREGON

Criminal homicide constitutes manslaughter in the second degree when: ...a person intentionally causes or aids another person to commit suicide. (ORS, Section 163.125.)

PENNSYLVANIA

A person who intentionally aids or solicits another to commit suicide is guilty of a felony of the second degree if his conduct causes such suicide or an attempted suicide, and otherwise of a misdemeanor of the second degree. (CPSA, Section 2505 (b))

SOUTH DAKOTA

Any person who intentionally in any manner advises, encourages, abets or assists another in taking his own life is guilty of a ...felony. (SDC, Section 22-16-37)

TEXAS

(a) A person commits an offense if, with intent to promote or assist the commission of suicide by another, he aids or attempts to aid the other to commit or attempt to commit suicide.

(b) An offense under this section is a class C misdemeanor unless the actor's conduct causes suicide or attempted suicide that results in serious bodily injury, in which event the offense is a felony of the third degree. (Texas Penal Code. Ann., Section 22.08)

WASHINGTON

A person guilty of promoting a suicide attempt when he knowingly causes or aids another person to attempt suicide. Promoting a suicide attempt is a ...felony. (RCW, Section 9A.36.060).

WISCONSIN

Whoever with intent that another take his or her own life assists such person to commit suicide is guilty of a ...felony. (Criminal Code, Section 940.12)

Derek Humphry writes: if you are a resident of a state not listed above, it merely means that possible prosecution could come under a more general law.

Michigan state Court of appeals in 1983 threw out murder charges against man who had obtained a gun and ammunition, then left them with a depressed friend who shot himself. Saying that aiding suicide is not against the law in Michigan, the court added: "The Legislature has not defined aiding suicide as crime, aiding a suicide does not fall within any definitions of homicide". (Lansing State Journal, March 23, 1983.)

THE HEMLOCK MANIFESTO

TOWARDS ACCEPTING VOLUNTARY EUTHANASIA

A set of guiding principles which should be included in right-to-die legislatio

Offered for consideration by

**The HEMLOCK SOCIETY, Supporting the Option
of Active Voluntary Euthanasia for the Terminally Ill**

The ideas and statements in this document are offered for consideration an debate in order to advance the cause of active voluntary euthanasia, also know as self-deliverance. The principles and draft directives do not represent Hemlock final position on the subject, and are offered for consideration by all.

Suggestions for improvements to this document will be welcome. Please sen to: Legal Panel, Hemlock Society, P.O. Box 66218, Los Angeles, Californi 90066.

1. **General Principles**

   a. It is not criminal in any way, nor is it evidence of mental instability c incompetence, nor is it unethical or immoral, for anyone to plan to c attempt to terminate his/her own life.

   b. If a person is known to have held the philosophy of voluntary euthanasi and/or has been a member of a right-to-die group, and/or has execute a living will, and has appointed a named person to make life or deat decisions for him/her that person may make any such decision tha he/she himself/herself could have made if he/she had retained his/h ability to decide.

   c. **Assistance provision**

      A. ''Terminal illness' means that the person is likely, in the judgmer of two examining physicians, to die of that condition within s months.

      B. Incurable distress is a legally insufficient basis for justification unle it is a product of terminal illness.

      C. It is not criminal in any way, nor is it wrongful legally, professiona ly or socially, for a medical doctor to withhold or terminate trea ment designed to extend the life of a terminally ill person who ha expressed opposition to such treatment in a legally relevant way

D. It is a breach of professional duty for a medical doctor in charge of the treatment of a terminally ill person who has demanded in a legally relevant way that his/her life not be extended by commencing or continuing treatment solely or primarily designed for that purpose not to respect that demand or promptly to arrange a transfer of responsibility to one who will.

E. It is not criminal in any way, nor is it wrongful legally, or socially for any relative or next friend to be present and/or to offer solace and encouragement to a person who has chosen to end his/her life, and who at that time or later does do so.

F. It is a breach of duty for anyone who has control in fact of a terminally ill person who has requested or demanded in a legally relevant way that his/her life not be extended by commencing or continuing treatment solely or primarily designed for that purpose not to respect that demand or promptly to arrange a transfer of control to one who will.

G. It is not criminal in any way, nor is it wrongful legally, professionally, or socially, for a medical doctor to provide moral support, aid or the instrumentality to accelerate the death of a terminally ill patient who has requested or demanded that cooperation in a legally relevant way.

H. It is a breach of professional duty for a medical doctor or other health care professional in charge of the treatment of a terminally ill patient who has requested or demanded in a legally relevant way that (s)he be provided with assistance in accelerating his/her death not to inform other concerned persons of that wish.

I. It is a breach of duty for anyone who has control in fact of a terminally ill person who has requested or demanded in a legally relevant way that (s)he be provided assistance in accelerating his/her death not to inform other concerned persons of that wish.

J. A legally cognizable declaration may be made:

    1. Writing—Any person of sufficient capacity to understand the significance of his/her conduct, regardless of age or other considerations, may execute a declaration directing the withholding or withdrawal of life sustaining procedures from themselves should they be in a terminal condition. The declaration should be: (1) in writing or other permanent form; (2) signed or authenticated by the person making it or by another in the declarant's presence at his/her direction; (3) dated; and (4) signed or authenticated by two or more witnesses to the execution. [Witness may not be: (1) one who signed declaration at behest of declarant; (2) related to declarant by blood or marriage; (3) entitled to any part of estate

101

of declarant, whether by statute or will; directly, financially responsible for declarant's medical care; or (4) the attending physician, an employee of the attending physician, or an employee of a health care facility in which declarant is a patient.]

[(a) copy to be provided at instance of declarant to attending physician. (b) physician to make declaration part of medical records of patient.]

(c) Revocation. (A) "A declaration may be revoked by burning, tearing or otherwise defacing it by or at instance of declarant with the intent to revoke; (B) by oral expression of desire to revoke, in the presence of a witness [as described above].]

[(d) duty to notify attending physicians is on declarant (e) physician to incorporate into medical record (f) physician to certify terminal condition and record in medical record, then inform patient or someone in his/her behalf that he/she is now governed by the declaration or revocation.]

2. Any person suffering a condition [described above] may declare in writing or in other permanent form [as described above] a wish to accelerate his/her own death through the positive intervention of his/her attending physician, after consultation with another physician as to declarant's condition and its intractibility. Such physician shall not be liable criminally, civilly, professionally or socially if he/she provides the assistance required. If he/she is unable or unwilling to do so, the patient must be transferred to another physician who is willing.

[(a) A husband, wife, child, grandchild, parent or grandparent, or other close relative, or next friend, who provides such assistance under similar safeguards also shall be held faultless.]

K. These principles involve the repeal of criminality for some assisted suicides. In those instances where the conditions are not complied with, the law of criminal homicide should control. [No special statute dealing solely with suicides should be enacted. (a) In sympathetic cases, (A) prosecutors are less likely to prosecute, and (B) jurors are less likely to convict, than if the crime "sounds" less serious. (C) "Maliciously assisting a suicide" being a "new crime," will not necessarily have all the safeguards against unfair conviction that the common law has developed for criminal homicide prosecutions.]

L. The declaration, if not in writing, should be sufficient to convey the same message and be safeguarded as nearly similarly as consistent with the medium used.

SUGGESTED LEGAL DOCUMENTS

The Hemlock Society is not engaged in the practice of law, nor do we purport to give legal advice. Therefore, if you propose to use any one of the following documents, we strongly urge that you contact an attorney for advice.

THE DURABLE POWER OF ATTORNEY
For Health Care

An Introduction

An important development in recent California law takes an old idea from business and commerce and adapts it to self-regulation of dying. Agency involves the appointment of someone you trust to make decisions for you. For hundreds of years it has been possible to give someone else the power to sell your house or buy a boat for you. Normally that power of representation terminates if its creator becomes incompetent through insanity or otherwise. However, in response to that problem, legal forms were devised expressing the intent to prevent that from occurring — to cause the "Power of Attorney" (agency) to survive the inability of the principal to decide things personally.

There is good reason to believe that the power effectively to get an agent whose decision-making powers survive the on-set of incompetence in the principal applies equally to health and life decisions. However, just to be sure the California legislature (Senate Bill 762) has put any lingering doubts to rest by passing a statute making it so.

In the inimitable fashion of lawyers, the term "Durable Power of Attorney" has been coined to express the idea that an appointment of another document, appropriately phrased, may continue in effect even when its creator is unable to make such decisions — the time, of course, when a terminal patient may need it most.

We cannot, therefore, give assurance that any of these documents will have particular legal effect in any state or country. However, should you desire to order your affairs in this manner you certainly can do no harm — and may do a great deal of good — by asking a lawyer to prepare some such document or documents for your signature.

WARNING TO PERSON EXECUTING
THIS DOCUMENT
(California Civil Code Sections 2410-2433)

This is an important legal document. It creates a durable power of attorney for health care. Before executing this document, you should know these important facts:

1. This document gives the person you designate as your attorney in fact the power to make health care decisions for you, subject to any limitations or statement of your desires that you include in this document. The power to make health care decisions for you may include consent, refusal of consent, or withdrawal of consent to any care, treatment, service, or procedure to maintain, diagnose, or treat a physical or mental condition. You may state in this document any types of treatment or placements that you do not desire.

2. The person you designate in this document has a duty to act consistently with your desires as stated in this document or otherwise made known or, if your desires are unknown, to act in your best interests.

3. Except as you otherwise specify in this document, the power of the person you designate to make health care decisions for you may include the power to consent to your doctor not giving treatment or stopping treatment which would keep you alive.

4. Unless you specify a shorter period in this document, this power will exist for seven years from the date you execute this document and, if you are unable to make health care decisions for yourself at the time when this seven-year period ends, this power will continue to exist until the time when you become able to make health care decisions for yourself.

5. Notwithstanding this document, you have the right to make medical and other health care decisions for yourself so long as you can give informed consent with respect to the particular decision. In addition, no treatment may be given to you over your objection, and health care necessary to keep you alive may not be stopped if you object.

6. You have the right to revoke the appointment of the person designated in this document by notifying that person of the revocation orally or in writing.

7. You have the right to revoke the authority granted to the person designated in this document to make health care decisions for you by notifying the treating physician, hospital, or other health care provider orally or in writing.

8. The person designated in this document to make health care decisions for you has the right to examine your medical records and to consent to their disclosure unless you limit this right in this document.

9. If there is anything in this document that you do not understand, you should ask a lawyer to explain it to you. This power of attorney will not be valid for making health care decisions unless it is either (1) signed by two qualified

witnesses who are personally known to you and who are present when you sign or acknowledge your signature or (2) acknowledged before a notary public in California.

A Durable Power of Attorney
For Health Care

To my family, relatives, my friends, my physicians, health care providers, community care facilities, and any other person who may have an interest or duty:

Appointment made this _____ day of _____ 198_____

at _____
(address)

I, _____ ,
(Full name)

being of sound mind, freely, willfully and voluntarily hereby appoint

_____ of _____ ,
(full name of attorney in fact/proxy)   (address)

Telephone number _____ as my attorney in fact/proxy to make health care decisions in my stead and behalf. He/she is not a treating health care provider nor an employee of such, nor is she/he an operator of a community health care facility which is treating me, or an employee of such, nor is he/she conservator of my person or estate; and I hereby request that he/she never be appointed such a conservator.

At any time I should for any reason be unable to make such decisions for myself, I hereby authorize

_____
(full name of attorney in fact/proxy)

my attorney-in-fact, to make any decisions I otherwise could make involving consent, refusal of consent, or withdrawal of consent to any care, treatment, service, or procedure to maintain, diagnose, or treat me for any physical or mental condition whatever, except for commitment to or placement in a mental health treatment facility, convulsive treatment, psychosurgery, sterilization or abortion.

This appointment shall have no legal force or effect after expiration of seven years from the date of its execution. It shall have no effect if I revoke it by giving notice of such revocation either orally or in writing.

(If you are not a resident of California, strike first sentence out. If a resident of California, see notice on reverse side of this paper.)

This document revokes any prior Durable Power of Attorney for Health Care.

SPECIAL PROVISIONS AND LIMITATIONS

If there is any type of treatment or placement that you do not want your attorney-in-fact to consent to or other restrictions you wish to place on his/her authority, you should list them in the space below. If you do not write in any limitations, your attorney-in-fact will have the broad powers to make health care decisions on your behalf which are included above.

In exercising authority under this Durable Power of Attorney, the authority of my attorney-in-fact is limited as stated below:

_____

_____

_____

_____

_____

STATEMENT OF DESIRES

Your attorney-in-fact must make decisions consistent with your known desires. You can, <u>but are not required to,</u> indicate your desires below. If your desires are unknown, he/she must act in your best interests. A judicial proceeding may be necessary to determine what is in your best interests. To reduce the risk of the need for court proceedings, you may wish to initial the statement or statements below that reflect your desires and/or write your own statements in the space below.

(If the statement reflects your desires, initial the box next to the statement.)

1. I desire that my life **be prolonged** to the greatest extent possible, without regard to my condition, the chances I have for recovery or long term survival, or the cost of the procedures.   (_____)

2.   If I am in a coma which my doctors have resonable   (_____)
     concluded is irreversible, I desire that life-sustaining
     or prolonging treatments or procedures **not** be used.

3.   If I have an incurable or terminal condition or ill-   (_____)
     ness and no reasonable hope of long term recovery
     or survival, I desire that life sustaining or prolonging
     treatments **not** be used.

4.   In deciding any questions under this document, my   (_____)
     attorney-in-fact is to consider the relief of suffering,
     the preservation or restoration of functioning, and
     the quality as well as the possible extension of my life.

OTHER OR ADDITIONAL STATEMENTS OF DESIRES

_____

_____

_____

_____

_____

_____

_____

_____

DESIGNATION OF ALTERNATE ATTORNEY-IN-FACT

You may wish to designate an alternative attorney-in-fact, in case the attorney-in-fact designated is unable or unwilling to act. NOTE: If the attorney-in-fact is your spouse, his/her authority automatically terminates if you are divorced.

If the person designated as my attorney-in-fact is unable or unwilling to make health care decisions for me, the following person shall serve in his/her place:

Name _____

Address_____

Telephone Number _____

BEFORE SIGNING YOU MUST READ THE WARNING TO PERSON EXECUTING THIS DOCUMENT (Printed in full at the start of this document.)

Signed _____

City, County and State of Residence_____

_____

_____

Date _____

TWO WITNESSES
(Document may be notarized instead)

I declare under penalty of perjury under the laws of California,[1]_____

(other state)

that the principal who signed or acknowledged this **Durable Power of Attorney for Health Care Decisions** in my presence is known to me personally; that she/he appears to be of sound mind and to be under no duress, fraud, or undue influence; that I am not the person appointed as attorney in fact by this document; that I am not a health care provider, an employee of a health care provider, the operator of a community care facility, nor an employee of a community care facility. I am not related to the principal by blood, marriage, or adoption; and to the best of my knowledge, I am not entitled to any part of the estate of the principal upon her/his death either under a will now existing or by operation of law.[2]

Date _____ Witness _____

Address _____

SPECIAL REQUIREMENTS

For persons who are patients in skilled nursing facilities in California/other state.

The principal is a patient in a skilled nursing facility in California[3]_____

(other state)

_____ as defined in subdivision (c) of Section 1250 of the

(other state)

Health and Safety Code of California[3] at the time she/he executed this document. Therefore, and in order to make it legally effective in California[3] _____ I _____ ,

(other state)   (full name of witness)

a patient - advocate/an ombudsman[4] as designated by the State Department of Aging[3] or other duly authorized person, am serving as a witness pursuant to section 2432 (f) of the California Civil Code.[5] _____

I declare under the penalty of perjury under the laws of California[3] _____ :

_____ I am not the person appointed as attorney in

(other state)

fact/proxy by this document; that I am not a health care provider, an employee of a health care provider, the operator of a community care facility, nor an employee of a community care facility; that I am not related to the principal by blood, marriage or adoption; and to the best of my knowledge I am not entitled to any part of the estate of the principal under a will now existing or by operation of law.

Date _____ Witness _____

Address _____

NOTARY

(Signer of instrument may either have it witnessed as above or have his/her signature notarized as below, to legalize this instrument.)

State of California _____

(Other State)

County of _____ ss

On this _____ day of _____ 198 _____

before me personally appeared _____

(full name of signer of instrument)

to me known (or proved to me on basis of satisfactory evidence.) to be the peron whose name is subscribed to this instrument, and acknowledged that he/she executed it. I declare under penalty of perjury that the person whose name is subscribed to this instrument appears to be of sound mind and under no duress, fraud or undue influence.

NOTARY SEAL   _____

(Signature of Notary)

FOOTNOTES

1. Strike out California and insert name of state where the principal (signer of this instrument) resides.
2. Under the law of California only one of the two witnesses must satisfy this last requirement. However, it is advisable to have both satisfy it.
3. If not a resident of California, strike out this term and add an appropriate alternative term. Although any other state may have no such requirement, it would do no harm to take the precaution of having the additional witness described in this paragraph.
4. Strike out the term which is inapplicable.

THE LIVING WILL: AN INTRODUCTION

The "Living Will" document on the next page conforms to the laws of California and would probably be respected by courts in other states. The following 21 states have their own Natural Death Acts: Alabama, Arkansas, Delaware, Florida, Georgia, Washington D.C., Idaho, Illinois, Kansas, Mississippi, Nevada, New Mexico, North Carolina, Oregon, Texas, Vermont, West Virginia, Virginia, Washington, and Wisconsin and Wyoming. If you require copies please send a number 10 (legal size) self-addressed, stamped envelope to: The Society for the Right to Die, 250 W. 57th St., New York, NY 10107.

A Living Will

A directive to withhold treatment and for the administration of pain-killing drugs

To my family, my relatives, my friends, my physicians, my employers, and all others whom it may concern:

Directive made this _____ day _____ 198____

I, _____ (name), being of sound mind, willfully, and voluntarily make known my desire that my life shall not be prolonged artificially under the circumstances set forth below, do hereby declare:

1. If at any time I should have an incurable injury, disease, illness or condition certified to be terminal by two medical doctors who have examined me, and where the application of life-sustaining procedures of any kind would serve only to prolong artificily the moment of my death, and where a medical doctor determines that my death is imminent, whether or not life-sustaining procedures are utilized, I direct that such procedures be withheld or withdrawn and that I be permitted to die naturally, and that I receive whatever quantity of whatever drugs may be required to keep me free of pain or distress even if the moment of death is hastened.

2. In the absence of my ability to give directions regarding the use of life-sustaining procedures, I hereby appoint _____

_____ (NAME) currently residing at _____

_____ , as my attorney in fact/proxy for the making of decisions relating to my health care in my place; and it is my intention that this appointment shall be honored by him/her, by my family, relatives, friends, physicians and lawyer as the final expression of my legal right to refuse medical or surgical treatment; and I accept the consequences of such a decision. I have duly executed a Durable Power of Attorney for health care decisions on this date.*

3. In the absence of my ability to give further directions regarding my treatment, including life-sustaining procedures, it is my intention that this directive shall be honoured by my family and physicians as the final expression of my legal right to refuse or accept medical and surgical treatment, and I accept the consequences of such refusal.

4. If I have been diagnosed as pregnant and that diagnosis is known to any interested person, this directive shall have no force during the course of my pregnancy.

5. I have been diagnosed, and notified at least 14 days ago, as being in a terminal condition by _____, M.D., whose address is _____ and whose telephone number is _____ . I understand that if I have not filled in the physician's name and address, it shall be presumed that I did not have a terminal condition when I made out this directive.**

6. This directive shall have no force and effect after five years from the date (above) of its execution, nor, if sooner, after revocation by me, either orally or in writing.

7. I understand the full importance of this directive and am emotionally and mentally competent to make this directive. No participant in the making of this directive or in its being carried into effect, whether it be a medical doctor, my

spouse, a relative, friend or any other person shall be held responsible in any way, legally, professionally or socially, for complying with my directions.

Signed _____

City, County and State _____

of residence _____

_____

_____

The declarant has been known to me personally and I believe her/him to be of sound mind.

Witness _____

address _____

Witness _____

address _____

Footnotes:

* Under California law, for such an appointment to be as fully effective as the law will permit, it must be in the form included on next page under the title "DURABLE POWER OF ATTORNEY FOR HEALTH CARE DECISIONS." Persons living in other states and executing this "Living Will" also might wish to execute that form (Durable Power of Attorney), as it might be honored by the courts of any particular state.

** If you are not a resident of California, strike out paragraph 5 in its entirety.

This directive complies in form with the Natural Death Act, California Health and Safety Code.

APPENDIX D

THE WORLD MOVEMENT

Organizations throughout the world which are concerned with right-to-die issues. Inclusion in this list does not necessarily mean that the group believes in active voluntary euthanasia; some accept only the principle of passive euthanasia.

Australia

West Australia V E S
P.O. Box 7243 Cloisters SQ, Perth 6000, WA, Australia
V E S of Victoria
P.O. Box 71 Mooroolbark Victora, Australia, 3138
V E S of N S W
P.O. Box 25 Broadway 2007, New South Wales, Australia

Belgium

A D M D Belgique
Rue de la Pastorale 84, 1080 Brussels, Belgium

Britain

Voluntary Euthanasia Society (Formerly EXIT)
13 Prince of Wales Terrace, London, W8 5 PG.
Voluntary Euthanasia Society of Scotland
17 Hart St., Edinburgh EHI 3RO, Scotland UK

Canada

(East Canada)
Dying with Dignity
P.O. Box 232, Station z, Toronto Ontario M5N 2Z4
(West Canada)
Dying with Dignity
301-2130 West 3rd Ave., Vancouver B.C. V6K 1L1

Colombia

Fundacion Pro Derecho a Morir Dignamente (D.M.D.)
Apartado Aereo 89314, Bogota DE Colombia, South America

Denmark

MIT Livstestamente
Ordrup Jagtvej 55, CharLotten Lund 2920, Denmark

France

ADMD
92 Bd. du Port Royal, 75005 Paris, France

Germany

D.G.H.S.
Postfach   11 05 29, 8900 Augsburg, West Germany

Holland

N.V.V.V.E.

Postbus 5331, 1007 AH Amsterdam, Netherlands

S.V.E.

Postbus 85843, 2508 CM The Hague, The Netherlands

I.C.V.E.

Zuiderweg 42   8993 KT, Vinkega, The Netherlands

India

Society for Right to Die With Dignity

Manackjee Wadia Bdg. 4th fl., 127 Mahatma Gandhi Rd.

Fort Bombay 400-001 India

Japan

Japan Society for Dying With Dignity

Hamaso Bld. 1-11, Ogawa Machi Kanada Chijoda Ku, Tokyo, Japan 101

New Zealand

Voluntary Euthanasia Society (Wellington)

95 Melrose Rd., Island Bay Wellington 2, New Zealand

V E Society (Auckland) Inc.

40 Willcott St., Mount Albert 3 Auckland, New Zealand

South Africa

S.A.V.E.S.

P.O. Box 37141, Overport 4067 Durban, South Africa

Spain

Asociacion Derecho a Morir Dignamente (D.M.D.) Apartado 9094 Madrid, 28080 Espana

Sweden

R.T.V.D.

Linnegatan 7, 114 47 Stockholm, Sweden

Switzerland

EXIT (German speaking)

Limmattalstrasse 177, CH 8049, Zurich

EXIT — A D M D (French speaking)

P.O. Box 100, 1222 Vesenaz, Geneva, Switzerland

U.S.A.

Concern for Dying

250 West 57th St., New York, NY 10107

Hemlock Society

P.O. Box 66218, Los Angeles, Ca 90066

Society for the Right to Die

250 West 57th St., New York, NY 10107

BIBLIOGRAPHY

This selected bibliography is set out in an unorthodox manner so that those wishing to read further can pick their books by the categories which most appeal to them. It is not an exhaustive list but comprises the books we have found the most useful. For the benefit of our overseas readers, where known, we have given the publishers in other countries. Do not assume because no publisher other than the U.S.A. is given that there is not one.

Advisory

Dealing Creatively with Death: A Manual of Death Education and Simple Burial, by Ernest Morgan, 10th edition, (The Celo Press, 1901 Hannah Branch Rd., Burnsville, North Carolina 28714, 1984, $8.50 incl. postage/packing)

Counseling the Dying, by Bowers et al (Harper and Row, 1981)

Let The Patient Decide. A Doctor's Advice to Older Persons, by Louis Shattuck Baer, M.D., (The Westminister Press, Philadelphia, 1978)

Concerning Death: A Practical Guide for the Living. Edited by Earl A. Grollman, (Beacon Press, Boston, 1974)

On Dying With Dignity, by Patrick F. Sheely, M.D., (Pinnacle, 1981)

Case Histories

Assisted Suicide: The Compassionate Crime, (Hemlock Society, $4)

Act of Love, by Paige Mitchell, (Bantam Paperbacks, 1977)

Death Be Not Proud: A Memoir, by John Gunther, (Perennial Library, 1965)

Gerhard: A Love Story, by Betty Kennedy, (Totem Books, Toronto, 1976)

Jean's Way, by Derek Humphry with Ann Wickett, (Quartet Books: London and New York; Fontana paperbacks, British Commonwealth, 1978; Available from Hemlock, $6)

Jeanette: A Memoir, by Tom Brown, (Lester and Orpen, Toronto, 1978)

Death of a Man, by L. Wertenbaker, (Random House, New York, 1957)

Exit House: Choosing Suicide as an Alternative, by Jo Roman, (Seaview Books, New York, 1980)

A Private Battle, by Cornelius Ryan and Kathryn Morgan Ryan, (Fawcett Popular Library, New York, 1980)

Karen Ann. The Quinlans Tell Their Story, by Joseph and Julia Quinlan with Phyllis Battelle, (Bantam Books, New York, 1977)

Endings and Beginnings, by Sandra H. Albertson. (Random House, 1980)

Facing Death Personally

Anatomy of an Illness as Perceived by the Patient, by Norman Cousins, (W.W. Norton, New York, 1979)

In the Company of Others, by Jory Graham. (Harcourt Brace Jovanovich, 1982)

First You Cry, by Betty Rollin, (Signet, New York, 1977)

Do Not Go Gentle, by Herbert M. Howe, (W.W. Norton, New York, 1980)

Voices of Death. Letter, Diaries and Other Personal Documents From People Facing Death that Prove Comforting Guidance for Each of us, by Edwin Shneidman, (Harper and Row, New York, 1980)

Stay of Execution: A Sort of Memoir, by Stewart Alsop, (J.B. Lippincott, New York, 1973)

Heartsounds, by Martha W. Lear. (Pocket Books, 1980)

Euthanasia

Euthanasia and the Right to Death, edited by A.B. Downing, (Peter Owen: London, Humanitites Press: New York, 1969)

Morals and Medicine, by Joseph Fletcher, (Beacon Press, Boston, 1954)

Good Life, Good Death: A Doctor's Case for Euthanasia and Suicide, by Christiaan Barnard, M.D., (Prentice Hall, New York, 1980)

Causing Death and Saving Lives, by Jonathan Glover, (Penguin Books, New York and London, 1978)

Whose Life Is It Anyway?, a play by Brian Clark, (Avon, New York, 1980)

Dying, by John Hinton. (Penguin, London, 1967)

Freedom to Die: Moral and Legal Aspects of Euthanasia, by O. Ruth Russell, revised edition, (Human Sciences Press, New York and London, 1977)

Death Without Dignity: Killing for Mercy, by Reverend Paul Marx, O.S.B., (The Liturgical Press, Collegeville, Minnesota, 1978)

Death by Choice, by Daniel C. Maguire (Schocken Books, 1975)

Suicide

Commonsense Suicide: The Final Right, by Doris Portwood, (Dodd, Mead, New York, 1978; Hemlock Society, Paperback, 1983, $8)

The Savage God. A Study of Suicide, by A. Alvarez, (Bantam Books, 1976)

Suicide: A Study in Sociology, by Emile Durkheim, (Free Press Paperback, Macmillan, 1966)

Suicide. The Philosophical Issues, edited by M. Pabst Battin and David J. Mayo, (St. Martin's Press, New York, 1980)

Ethical Issues in Suicide, by M. Pabst Battin (Prentice-Hall, 1982)

Suicide and Ethics, by M. Pabst Battin and Ronald W. Maris (Human Sciences Press, New York, 1983)

Grief

Grief and How To Live With It, by Sarah Morris, (Grosset and Dunlap, New York, 1972)

Learning to Say Goodby. When a Parent Dies, by Eda LeShan, (Avon, New York, 1978)

Widow, by Lynn Caine, (Bantam Books, 1975)

Facing Death and Grief, by George N. Marshall, (Prometheus Books, 1981)

Hospice

A Way To Die, by Victor and Rosemary Zorza, (Alfred A. Knopf, New York, 1980)

Hospice. Creating New Models of Care for the Terminally Ill, by Parker Rossman, (Fawcett Columbine, New York, 1980)

The Hospice Movement. A Better Way of Caring for the Dying, by Sandol Stoddard, (Stein and Day, New York, 1978)

Quest: The Life of Elisabeth Kubler-Ross, by Derek Gill, (Harper and Row, New York, 1980)

To Live Until We Say Goodbye, Text by Elisabeth Kubler-Ross; photographs by Mal Warshaw, (Prentice Hall, New Jersey, 1978)

Novels

Love Story, by Erich Segal, (Coronet Books, Hodder and Stoughton, 1971)

In the Night Season, by Christiaan Barnard, (Prentice Hall, New Jersey, 1978)

The Woman Said Yes, by Jessamyn West, (Harcourt, Brace, Jovanovich, 1976)

Toxicology

The Pharmacological Basis of Therapeutics, by Goodman and Gilman, 6th edition, (Macmillan, New York, 1980)

Clinical Toxicology of Commercial Products, by Gosselin, Hodge, Smith, and Gleason, 4th edition, (Williams and Wilkins, Baltimore, 1979)

Toxicology: the Basic Science of Poisons, by Cassarett and Doull, 2nd edition, (Macmillan, New York, 1980)

The Use and Misuse of Sleeping Pills. A Clinical Guide, by Wallace B.

Mendelson, M.D., (Plenum Medical Book Company, New York and London, 1980)

Physician's Desk Reference, 34th edition, (Medical Economics Company, New Jersey, 1980)

The Essential Guide to Prescription Drugs, by James W. Long, M.D., (Harper and Row, New York, 1980)

The Merck Manual, 13th edition, (Merck Sharp and Dohme Research Laboratories, New Jersey, 1980)

How to Die With Dignity, by George B. Mair, M.D., F.R.C.S., F.R.R.P., F.R.S.G.S. (Scottish Exit, Edinburgh, 1980)

The Prediction of Suicide, edited by Drs. Beck, Resnick and Lettieri, (The Charles Press, Philadelphia, 1974)

Justifiable Euthanasia, a manual for physicians, by Dr. P. V. Admiraal, (Netherlands Voluntary Euthanasia Society, Amsterdam, 1981)

Current Medical Diagnosis and Treatment, edited by Marcus A. Krupp, M.D., and Milton J. Chatton, M.D., (Lange Medical Publications, Los Altos, California, 1981)

Handbook of Poisoning, by Robert H. Dreisbach, M.D., Ph.d., 11th edition, (Lange Medical Publications, Los Altos, California, 1983)

Psychology of Death

Death: Current Perspectives, by Edwin S. Shneidman, 3rd edition, (Mayfield, Palo Alto, California, 1984)

Death. The Final Stage of Growth, by Elisabeth Kubler-Ross, (Prentice Hall, New Jersey, 1975)

The Denial of Death, by Ernest Becker, (Free Press: Macmillan, New York, 1973)

Facing Death, by Robert E. Kavanaugh, (Penguin Books, New York, 1976)

The Human Encounter With Death, by Stanislav Grof, M.D., and Joan Halifax, Ph.D., (E.P. Dutton, New York, 1977)

Life After Life, by Raymond Moody, Jr., M.D., (Bantam Books, 1977)

The Meaning of Death, edited by Herman Feifel, (McGraw-Hill Paperbacks New York, 1965)

On Death and Dying, by Elisabeth Kubler-Ross, (Macmillan, New York, 1976)

On Dying and Denying: A Psychiatric Study of Terminality, by Avery D Weisman, (Behavioral Publications Inc., New york, 1978)

Questions and Answers on Death and Dying, by Elisabeth Kubler-Ross, (Mac millan, New York, 1977)

The Way We Die. An Investigation of Death and Dying in America Today by David Dempsey, (McGraw-Hill, New York, 1977)

Surveys

Who Believes in Voluntary Euthanasia? (A survey of the membership of the Hemlock Society.) 1983, From Hemlock. $3, plus $1 postage.

APPENDIX E

xtracted from:

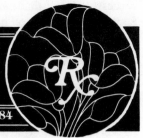

Hemlock Quarterly

litor: Ann Wickett   Issue 14: January 1984

Groups can discuss suicide in general: no involvements

y Curt Garbesi

There has been much interest lately among the membership, and particularly fter our conference in San Francisco, in the creation of mutual support groups ɔ help deal especially with crisis situations. This, of course, is a laudable ac-vity, since we have within our group incomparable human resources for pro-iding each other with companionship, comfort, and aid. However, there are ertain legal risks incident to such conduct of which you should be aware in rder to avoid potential problems.

Before discussing the dangers you may be facing, it should be stated that nere is literally nothing which the law excludes from simple discourse, at least ι the United States—the first amendment to the Constitution assures that. So, ɔ the extent that you only discuss, and only in general terms—not related to ny particular person or problem—there is no risk involved. It is also fair to ιy that particular people and their conditions are safely subject to discussion, ɔ long as the interchange is limited. It is the limitations that I want to convey.

I should add also that the risks that I describe here are not very likely to ιaterialize in any particular situation. Generally, any such support-group is erceived as providing an invaluable social service. Thus, police and rosecutors—and later, judges and juries—are not likely to be zealous in in-rfering with the people involved.

However, our euthaniasia activities do run counter to age-old taboos and eeply-felt convictions of substantial numbers of our fellow citizens. They have egun to demonstrate their great power politically in recent years, and might vell be instrumental in initiating some kind of legal action, criminal or even ivil. So, at least we should be aware of the risks, no matter how slight, and void those in which we decide it is not necessary to engage.

The clearest violation of the criminal law would be if one person supplies nother with the instrumentality used for committing suicide. (Even the smallest ɘduction of life-span is significant.) In those jurisdictions, like California, where is a separate crime to "aid and abet" a suicide, such an act would at least iolate that law, subjecting the aider to a potentially substantial imprisonment ɘrm.

In California, the state might not be able to prosecute for criminal homicide successfully, but that question is still not clearly resolved. There is a recent Supreme Court opinion holding that the sole survivor of an only partially successful suicide pact may only be convicted of aiding and abetting a suicide—not murder.

Open Question

Whether that decision would be extended to include a case where the aide was not himself intending suicide is an open question. In at least some other jurisdictions, there is a risk of prosecution for murder or manslaughter. So if you want to avoid that possibility, however remote, DON'T provide poison or any other instrumentality, intended for use in committing suicide. If it is used successfully, you could be found guilty of aiding and abetting a suicide or even murder. If unsuccessful you might be prosecuted for an attempt to commit either crime. (Attempts are themselves criminal acts.)

Even the giving of advice or the urging of suicide can result in criminal liability. In some jurisdictions, including California, there would be no crime merely in the solicitation or advice itself. In some other states the result could be otherwise.

However, even in California—as well as other states—such advice followed by an actual suicide results in potentially severe punishment. So, to avoid such a possibility, DON'T advise, counsel or urge another to take his or her own life. It is more risky yet to urge a particularly described act designed to end a life.

Conspiracy

Yet more remote from an actual suicide, but raising substantial possibility of serious penal consequences is a "conspiracy" to "aid and abet" a suicide or to commit a homicide. If two or more people combine for the purpose of committing a crime, or even an "immoral act," and some act, however innocuous, is done in the furtherance of that plan, it is a serious crime in all jurisdictions. It doesn't matter that a death did not occur, or that it was not even attempted.

For example, if a group were to plan to encourage someone, whether a member of the group or not, to commit suicide, and anyone, pursuant to that understanding, bought a copy of a suicide manual, that would render all members of the group criminally liable for conspiracy. Legally, avoidance of this risk requires that groups of 2 or more persons not come to an understanding, tacit or explicit, that any one of them will even encourage some person to commit suicide, nor of course to assist in such an act. It should be noted that the act of encouraging, *etc.*, could occur during a meeting, and that might make the conspiracy complete.

There is additional risk which may be consequential upon there being a conspiracy in these situations. Those persons party to the conspiracy are also responsible criminally for any crime performed by any one of them in furtherance f their mutual understanding. This is even if the particular crime in question as not even adverted to in discussion in any way. It need only be a foreseeable onsequence of their having joined together as they did.

Thus, if any one of them provides the instrumentality for the commission f a suicide, all would be guilty of either attempting to aid and abet a suicide if a death actually ensued), or even of a criminal homicide, at least in some tates.

It is obvious, then, that conspiracy law dictates a great deal of circumspection in the conduct of support groups. (It should be noted here that the members eed not have ever actually met together in order to be found to have conspired. When Dr. Spock was tried during the Vietnam era, it was no defect in the prosecution's case that he had never even conversed with his co-defendants. It was sufficient that they all consciously sought the same illegal goal in support of each other.)

In addition to the risks of criminal prosecution there is also the problem of potential civil liability for damages. (The assumption in the following material is that anyone who is arguably liable criminally, on any theory, including conspiracy, could also be liable for damages.) The first situation to be considered ere is whether one who failed in an attempted suicide might recover against those who bungled in their assistance or advice, thereby causing the failure and possibly some new injury in the process.

If the subject were held to have been incompetent at the time of his attempt, it is possible that another found to have somehow induced or aided in the attempt could be held liable for any ensuing injuries caused by the attempt. (It is not probable that the costs of continued living would be compensable, however; it is difficult to imagine a court finding a duty to help in the ending f a life. Absent such a duty, one could hardly be held liable for expenses incident solely to causing its continuance by failing to extinguish it.)

If, however, the subject were found to be competent at the time of the attempt, the problem becomes much more complex. At least the assister should not be responsible for injuries the risk of which the subject was equally able to appreciate and avoid. Of course, if the assister had, or purported to have pecial expertise (a doctor, nurse, pharmacist, etc.), it is highly probable that substantial percentage of the loss would be attributed to him/her.

If the aided or encouraged suicide is completed, the question becomes whether the heirs or other survivors of the deceased could recover from the assister. All states have laws under which recovery may be had against one whose conduct wrongfully caused a death. If, therefore, it is established that someone has contributed to causing a death under circumstances making that conduct wrongful—as it would be in most assisted suicide cases—certain close relatives are entitled to recover any damages recognized as compensable under local law.

125

In many cases damages would not be substantial, because the life of the suicide, had it continued, due to illnesss, advanced age or other condition, would not have been of great value either economically or physically to those around him. However, the risk of substantial damage awards does exist.

Inheritances

Another problem that should be noted here is the effect of having committed a homicide upon the otherwise right to an interest in the estate of the deceased, either by inheritance or by will. There is a general principle of law that a person should not be permitted to profit from his own wrong. At least in a fair number of jurisdictions, this has led to denying to one who intentionally caused the death any right to participate in a distribution of the estate

In conclusion, a possible but not very probable consequence of a functioning mutual support group dealing with questions of suicide of a member, friend or relative of a member is some form of criminal prosecution and possible conviction. Another is potential liability for a judgment for damages. Understanding those risks may well affect your choices about how actually to conduct yourselves when faced with the cry of distress of other human beings who need your support.

(Curt Garbesi is professor of law, Loyola Law School, Los Angeles, and legal consultant to the Hemlock Society.)

tracted from:

Hemlock Quarterly

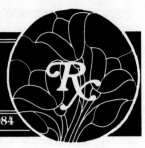

litor: Ann Wickett   Issue 14: January 1984

roup that dares not speak its name

y Doris Portwood

A New York discussion group, sometimes referring to itself as "hemlock" ith a small "h," dates from the spring of 1979. Seventeen area women who ad written to me about my book "Common-Sense Suicide" met to exchange ews on that subject. Later in the year, a number of people who wrote to Edard M. Brecher in support of his expressed views ("Opting for Suicide," NY imes Magazine, 3/18/79) met to form a second group of 15 to 20 women nd men. At the same time, a smaller group (possible 5 or 6) from Queens nd Long Island had one meeting. In time, the more active participants from iese groups, about 35 people, are notified of meetings; attendance varies from 5 to 25.

The group is completely unstructured: it has no officers, dues, base of operaons, address or telephone number. One "information person," as she has been lf-named, keeps a mailing list for the now-infrequent meetings that take place : some member's home.

Through the years, too, most members have come to know a few of the thers; any of us could, if necessary, make contact within the group. At one me, also, the membership was divided into 6-person "grids" whose grid leader ad phone numbers of the others and agreed to contact them for any signifiant reason. This grid arrangement has not so far been used.

Our New York group now meets only once a year. Most of the members ave a fair knowledge of methods and risks, of the legal situation, of the contiuing stigma, etc. Our main gain from the yearly meeting is the mutual comort that comes from a shared viewpoint on an often-evaded subject. What we ve in return is a commitment to support the destigmatizing of rational suicide, rough personal contact and media exposure, and the decriminalization of aid) a would-be suicide, through removal of legal restraints.

Kinship

With the advent of the Hemlock Society, as an open movement dedicated) similar goals, we discussed whether any need for our small discussion group remained. Suggestions to disband, however, met with near-unanimous opposi tion. Members expressed a strong feeling of kinship within the group and stress the "comfort" aspect of personal contacts. At the October (1983) meetin therefore, discussion turned on the possibility of becoming a Hemlock Socie chapter and we examined the 4-page "Do's and Don't's of Networking" th was sent out under Hemlock's covering letter of Oct. 4.

A few points from our group's experience may help other chapter-former Our own do's-and-don't's possibly over-accent the negative—but rememb that this effort dates back to 1979 when the climate was less accepting th now. We were breaking rather radical ground.

Our primary decision: we are *not* a mutual aid group. Our second: we a not an organization, and so cannot be spoken for by any individual. Thir we do not "advocate" either suicide or euthanasia; we discuss both, along wi other facets of living and dying. Negative or not, most of these decisions r main valid because the legal climate has not changed.

The media picture *has* altered dramatically (note Derek Humphry's full cale dar of TV and radio engagements in every part of the U.S. and Canada). T social climate, reflected in the media, is changing—but slowly.

Our group had to make an early decision about seeking or accepting publi ty. We received offers due, in part, to the fact that Jo Roman (author of *Ex House,* whose own planned suicide in 1979 was the subject of taped discussic used next year on TV) attended our first meeting.

She came as a stranger among strangers, like all of us. Newspaper interview TV and radio publicity were available to us but were rejected for the followir reasons: Several otherwise willing participants feared that public identificatic with such a cause would be detrimental to their jobs or careers. Others fear family opposition.

(Despite a professed dedication to removing the stigma associated with suicid we still have members who do not share with mates and/or offspring t knowledge of their group participation.) Our most "responsible" reason f refusing publicity, however, was and remains the fact that we have nothing offer to the people who, in response to the publicity, would seek to join su a group. We were unwilling to raise false hopes. (We still are not ready to e pand, but the Hemlock Society now offers a possible meeting-ground for pote tial new groups.)

Media queries

The media offers we have received are educational in that they reveal signi cant misconceptions about the likely members of a group such as ours. Inte viewers, who tend to be young and healthy, apparently see us as mainly o and decrepit. They may hesitantly ask, in a phone call, "Are many of yo — you know, uh, about ready to go?"

Several exploratory "offers" have come from producers looking for a fam ation to follow via TV. (This despite the wide adverse criticism of Jo Roman's t-arranged publicity.) Almost all such inquirers express surprise that we know no one currently planning a suicide.

In contrast to this picture, our members range in age from 40-up; their health oblems range from non-existent to serious; they are at least 80% women; ost are well educated and experienced and they have a diversity of interests i.e., they are not one-subject people. This fact is not entirely an asset: it ans that our "activists" often are also active in other fields as well. They ay not have time or inclination to, say, help new groups form or make trips local offices of representatives who might support right-to-die legislation, . We have agreed, in meeting, that we *should* offer help to any would-be w group; the carrying out of that chore might be less easy than our verbal reement.

Anonymous

All groups such as ours are likely to attract a few less-than-rational people. spite the care with which our members were originally contacted (all from *ir* letters of declared interest), after a third meeting-notice mailing one per- a wrote rather ominously that any further such mail would be called to the ention of the postal authorities. We accent and re-accent that no person is alified to speak in the name of the group. We have also agreed, however, at any person can speak or write about the group so long as individual onymity is respected and maintained.

The question of accessible meeting places presents some problems that might t affect a less "big city" group. At least half our membership (which in- des some New Jersey and Connecticut residents) live outside the immediate y. We may, in time, have to enlarge to the point where we can hire a public eting room or remain small enough to fit into the relatively few available y homes.

A possible future solution, if Hemlock forms chapters in this area, would to join together now and then (not more than annually) for an area meeting a public place. (Hemlock's 1981 and 1982 New York meetings each attracted some people; since their membership has increased by more than ten times the interim, a sizable and publicity-worthy New York meeting seems possible.) Our meetings are more than loosely put together, but interest does not wane d time often runs out before we realize it. We have had an "expert" or two ak to us, including one lawyer, and we always exchange any late news about ys and means. We call each other's attention to news items or feature ar- es and encourage members to write to editors, columnists and publishers, to call in to radio talk shows, with praise or criticism whenever "our topic" covered.

We discuss pending legislation, when there is any, and re-encourage each other contact our representatives and any relevant committees of federal or state government. We discuss recent developments in The Society for the Right to Die, Concern for Dying, Hemlock, the foreign euthanasia organizations and the World Federation of Right-to-Die Societies. We exchange information about book and article publication in the related fields, including patient's rights, living wills, etc.

Comfort and Laughter

Perhaps the most surprising thing about our group is its overall cheery tone. A tape of our first meeting is punctuated with laughter. Most who attend the meeting — cautiously, anxious, feeling a little worried — later express the feeling of relief and happiness that came of it.

Ours is not ghoulish laughter, as one young newspaper woman suggested might be. Most of us are relatively healthy but realistic people. Perhaps we have watched too much suffering on the part of a sick relative or visited too many friends in nursing homes. We can tell ourselves that with a little luck we'll skip that. We can be happy knowing we'll try to skip it, and relieved to meet many comradely people who feel the same way. Our jokes are not black humor — just plain humor pleasantly shared.

So — despite the negative factors that are stressed above — we all vote to continue to meet. Maybe we'll be a Hemlock chapter. At the least, we'll continue to give and receive mutual comfort.

Hemlock Quarterly is issued only to paid-up members. (Annual membership: $20.)

Other books from The Hemlock Society

(A non-profit educational corporation supporting the option of active voluntary euthanasia for the terminally ill.)

Commonsense Suicide: The Final Right
By Doris Portwood

An honest examination of the last taboo in our society.

$8.   Distributed by Grove Press
                                                     New York

Jean's Way
By Derek Humphry with Ann Wickett

The true story of one woman's plans to end her own life towards the end of a terminal illness. The book is helpful to other couples in a similar predicament. 1984 edition

$6.50   Distributed by Grove Press
                                                     New York

---

Assisted Suicide: The Compassionate Crime

A compilation of famous euthanasia cases from around the world. Invaluable as source material for researchers. Updated 1984.

$5 (includes mailing)   Only from The Hemlock Society

Who Believes in Voluntary Euthanasia?

A survey of Hemlock's membership in 1982. Important research data.

$4. (includes mailing)   Only from the Hemlock Society.
                                              P.O. Box 66218
                                           Los Angeles, CA 90066

THE HEMLOCK SOCIETY

A national organization, founded 1980, Los Angeles.
Non-profit, tax deductible 501c3

The Hemlock Society, an educational organization, supports the option of active voluntary euthanasia (self-deliverance) for the advanced terminally ill mature adult, or the seriously incurably physically ill person.

As suicide is no longer a crime, Hemlock believes that assistance in suicide should also be de-criminalized where a terminally ill or seriously incurably ill person requests this help.

If you have found yourself in general agreement with the principles of this book, you may wish to join the Hemlock Society for the following reasons:

1. To help the Society's campaign to bring better understanding of euthanasia and to work towards improved laws in this area.

2. To demonstrate through membership that you are in favour of thoughtful, justified, voluntary euthanasia for yourself.

3. To receive the Society's interesting quarterly newsletter, Hemlock Quarterly, to keep you up-to-date with ethical, legal and operating developments. This newsletter is the best informed on euthanasia in the world.

Annual membership (January through December)
$20.00 ($10.00 after July 1 each year.)

Donations to the Hemlock Society are tax-deductible.

THE HEMLOCK SOCIETY
PO BOX 66218
Los Angeles, CA 90066

Telephone: (213) 391-1871

LET ME DIE
BEFORE I WAKE

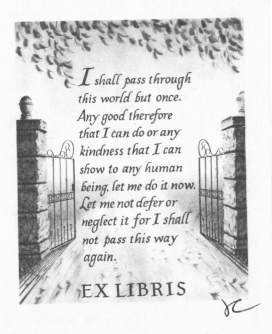

I shall pass through this world but once. Any good therefore that I can do or any kindness that I can show to any human being, let me do it now. Let me not defer or neglect it for I shall not pass this way again.

EX LIBRIS

TOM BRUCE